Menopause:
The One-Stop Guide

'This practical guide is a welcome addition to the range of material now available to help women understand their menopause. Kathy Abernethy is a highly qualified and experienced specialist nurse, greatly respected within the healthcare profession. She understands that menopause is an intensely personal experience, and offers thoughtful advice for treatment and lifestyle options.

'The book is especially helpful in providing clear definitions, answers to frequently asked questions and more than 200 anonymised quotes from patients expressing their concerns and anxieties during consultations at the author's clinical practice. This all gels into an easily digestible format that will inform, reassure and, as the title suggests, guide women through this inevitable stage of their lives.'

Medical Advisory Council,
The British Menopause Society

Kathy Abernethy works as part of an award-winning NHS menopause team in London and has a private clinic in south-west London. She holds a Master's in reproductive women's health, and speaks and writes regularly on the topic of menopause. She has written a book for nurses on menopause and HRT as well as numerous articles. Kathy raises awareness of the impact of menopause at work by delivering workplace sessions to staff and managers of various organisations throughout the UK, and in 2017 she was elected chair of the British Menopause Society, the leading professional organisation for the field, having been an active member since its inception in 1989.

Menopause:
The One-Stop Guide

*A practical guide to understanding and living
with the menopause*

Kathy Abernethy

P

PROFILE BOOKS

First published in Great Britain in 2018 by
PROFILE BOOKS LTD
3 Holford Yard
Bevin Way
London
WC1X 9HD

www.profilebooks.com

1 3 5 7 9 10 8 6 4 2

Designed and typeset by sue@lambledesign.demon.co.uk
Printed and bound by CPI Group (UK) Ltd, Croydon, CR0 4YY

The moral right of the author has been asserted.

The advice and recommendations given in this book are provided
in good faith, but no responsibility for any consequences, however
caused, of acting on them will be accepted by the author or the
publisher. If in doubt, seek suitable advice from a healthcare
professional.

A CIP catalogue record for this book is available from the
British Library.

ISBN 978 1 78125 872 9
eISBN 978 1 78283 366 6

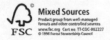

Mixed Sources
Product group from well-managed
forests and other controlled sources
www.fsc.org Cert no. TT-COC-002227
© 1996 Forest Stewardship Council
FSC

Contents

Introduction

How can you write a whole book on menopause? Isn't it a natural event, one that all women will eventually experience? As women, don't we know the signs and symptoms – changes in periods and hot flushes? Shouldn't we just get on with it? Well yes, many women do 'just get on with it', but in my many years of specialising in this area of health, I have met countless women who do not fully understand the changes that this time of hormone fluctuation can bring, or how long such symptoms may last. Yes, they all know about flushes and sweats, but many women worry about other symptoms, like mood changes, itching, tiredness, bladder symptoms and poor memory, not aware that these too can be linked to menopausal changes. In consultations with women, I spend a lot of time, saying 'yes, that's normal', as they take me through the often numerous symptoms they are experiencing. Women express their relief to have someone to talk to, someone to listen to their own particular experience of menopause and someone to guide them through the treatment options open to them. The women I see do not want to just walk out with a prescription; they want to understand the menopause, the effects it can have on the body and the different ways they might choose to help symptoms, both medical and non-medical.

Not all women have a 'normal' menopause, whatever we mean by that. Some will experience menopause suddenly, as a result of surgery or after treatment for cancer. Some may become menopausal by opting to have their ovaries removed in order to avoid cancer. Others will be very young, perhaps even still in their teens, when their ovaries stop working and so will have all the effects of early menopause. These women need support, information and treatment. For a few women, the symptoms of menopause will be very severe, affecting work, home and social life on a daily basis, sometimes for months or even years.

The women I see week in and week out tell me that no one has taken the opportunity to explain the changes and symptoms, discussed health after menopause, or explained that purposeful lifestyle changes around menopause can improve health well beyond menopause and even into old age. Some of the effects of menopause are inevitable, but others can be offset by positive lifestyle changes, for example to improve bone and heart health.

Menopause is no longer a taboo topic. In much of society (although, sadly, still not all), women will talk about menopause, whether it's the symptoms, the physical changes or the psychological effects it can sometimes have – you can read about it everywhere. The media has finally taken notice and some (still only a few) celebrities have been open about their own menopause experiences. There have been television and radio programmes about menopause and numerous women's magazines articles about it. Even the government has reported that women at work may be affected by menopause and the Chief Medical Officer, the most senior advisor on health matters to the government, has raised the topic, saying that menopause should be as freely discussed at work as any other health topic.

Yet, time and time again, women tell me that they have struggled to get help on a personal level; that they do not know which media stories to trust; and that GPs, while sympathetic, have little time to discuss the matter, or balance treatment options for them in a way that is meaningful. In short, women still feel alone at menopause, searching the internet and scouring leaflets to put together the information they need to make informed choices. This one-stop book on menopause aims to fill the gap, providing practical information about menopause, explaining what is normal and how you might choose to cope with it all. It will help you understand that there is more to the 'change of life' than simply stopping periods and aims to equip you to make positive choices at this important time. Throughout the text are anonymised quotes from real women who I have encountered in my clinical practice, and which express the kind of anxieties that many women have about going through the menopause.

Whether you see menopause as a natural event that does not need medical intervention, or whether you are open to all the medical help on offer, this book is for you.

chapter 1

Menopause

What is normal?

You would think as a woman I would know about these things, hormones and so on, but I really don't. No one prepares you.

In America, it is sometimes called the 'third talk': you know you get a talk on starting periods, one on sex and we need one on menopause!

As you approach your late forties, you are likely to be expecting that menopause will happen soon if it hasn't already. In the UK the average age of menopause is 51, so menopause usually happens when you are between the ages of 45 and 55. You would think, therefore, that it would not come as a shock, yet you may feel ill-prepared for it and surprised by the symptoms you experience. Unlike pregnancy, you won't find that friends raise the topic very often, or pass on books they have used or even give you their own tips and advice. Possibly they are going through it too, but it tends not to be 'coffee shop' talk. Even your mother will probably brush it off, saying that she doesn't remember or that it was 'no problem'. Look online, and you will see a huge amount of information. But what is reliable? What do you believe? Is it really that bad? What is normal?

Chapter 5 looks at what happens when women go through menopause much earlier than usual and the effects that an unusually early menopause can have. Young women going through menopause need specific and ongoing physical and psychological support, and that is discussed more in that chapter. But what about the so-called 'normal' woman? Is anything 'normal' about menopause? What can you expect and how do you know if anything is medically wrong with you or if it is just the natural progression of a normal life event?

I had these awful symptoms, and it made me wonder if I was actually sick; surely this is not normal?

We all know menopause can cause flushes and sweats, but everything else took me completely by surprise – the tiredness, feeling tearful and wondering if I would ever feel myself again.

If menopause is natural, why do I feel so awful? Surely I can do something about this?

What is menopause?

The term 'menopause' means different things to different people. To some, it simply explains the physiological change that occurs in a woman when periods stop and the ability to conceive is past. This conforms to the medical definition of menopause, which refers simply to the 'last menstrual bleed' or periods finally stopping. Using this definition, you cannot say you are 'menopausal' until this time has passed and, medically, once you have not had a period for one year, after the age of 50, you are deemed to be 'post-menopausal', meaning after menopause has happened. This time of hormonal change, though, is often accompanied by physical and psychological effects, which may start some time before periods finally stop and continue for a long time afterwards. These are 'menopausal symptoms' even though you may not fit the medical definition of actually being 'menopausal': that is, you can sometimes recognise that the menopause is starting before your doctor can confirm the diagnosis. It is for this reason that medical diagnosis of menopause should be based on your history and symptoms and not simply on blood tests. In fact, blood test results can confuse the diagnosis, as I will discuss later.

Pre-, peri-, post-menopause – what's the difference?

I feel as if I have been peri-menopausal for years.

You will find it helpful to understand how healthcare professionals describe menopause, so here are some common terms. These terms apply to women going through menopause at the usual time, i.e. around the age of 50. Younger women are described differently (see Chapter 5).

Menopause – the last ever period you have. Of course, you do not know it was the last period until some time after it has happened. Will there be another? Periods don't usually stop suddenly; more often they get gradually shorter and further apart until eventually they stop altogether. Medically, menopause is diagnosed retrospectively, one year after periods have stopped.

Peri-menopause – the months or even years before periods stop when hormonal changes start, and symptoms often occur. The peri-menopause continues until you are considered 'post-menopausal', that is for one year after your periods stop. The term covers the time leading up to your last period when hormonal changes start, when you may get symptoms, and then for the year afterwards. Peri-menopause can last a long time, with some women saying that they can feel the very start of menopausal changes in their late thirties, even though periods may be unchanged for several years after that.

Post-menopausal – when you have not had a natural period for one year. Once it has been twelve months since you have had a period, you are 'post-menopausal' from a medical perspective. If you are under 45, however, this diagnosis may not be as clear-cut, as there can be other reasons why periods stop in younger women.

My blood tests led my doctor to say I was not yet menopausal, but I had all the typical symptoms; it was very confusing to me.

Once you understand this terminology, you can begin to see why misunderstandings occur between women and their clinicians. Some doctors may say 'you are not menopausal' when what they mean is that there is no sign that your periods are stopping. It is not to say that the symptoms you are experiencing cannot be due to the hormonal changes of menopause, just that as yet your periods have not reflected the hormonal changes and finally stopped. Similarly, if you are described as being 'post-menopausal', you may think that that marks the end of these symptoms, but you may go on to have symptoms for a long time after you are described as 'post-menopausal'.

I can begin to see why it's called 'the change'.

Women themselves often use more accurate terminology. You might describe yourself as 'in the throes of menopause' or 'in the change', which describes more accurately what you are experiencing. The term 'peri-menopause' is much better understood too as it covers the wide time span when you might be getting symptoms, regardless of what is happening to your periods. The peri-menopause builds up towards the menopause and is followed eventually by post-menopause. The time this takes varies between individuals and might be a couple of years or several.

Why it happens

Back to biology, at least a bit. When you have a period, it is an indication that the 'menstrual cycle' is working. It does not necessarily mean that you can fall pregnant, as that requires a whole lot of other factors as well. The menstrual cycle ensures that the womb is ready to receive a pregnancy if it happens and, if it doesn't, the cycle repeats. Ovaries play a major role in releasing oestrogen, which influences the lining of the womb to grow and shed, which in turn leads to monthly periods. The hypothalamus, located in the brain, stimulates the pituitary nearby to release the hormones that tell the ovaries to release oestrogen, which then circulates through the body. When the ovaries are working properly, the messenger system between the ovaries and the pituitary generally works well. Once the ovaries have done their job that month and released enough oestrogen, the pituitary recognises that and switches off the messenger hormones until the next cycle. So, simply put, in a normal cycle you will see the rise of FSH, follicle stimulating hormone (the messenger), resulting in the ovaries producing oestrogen, then the fall in follicle stimulating hormone as the oestrogen rises. In the second half of the cycle, progesterone is produced ready to support a fertilised egg. If pregnancy does not occur, the progesterone hormone falls and that causes a period as the womb lining is shed for another month. There are many other hormones involved too, but, when thinking about menopause, these are the principle ones that are important. As you approach menopause, the ovaries cannot work efficiently because of ageing follicles (within the ovary) and your body cannot make new ovaries or follicles. This results in a fall in oestrogen over time until after the menopause when it remains very low unless you use hormone replacement therapy. At the same time, FSH, follicle stimulating hormone, gradually rises in response to low oestrogen levels.

So do I need hormone tests to diagnose menopause?

A simple blood test, just to confirm what I already suspect, would be really helpful.

My doctor said this couldn't be menopause because my blood tests don't confirm it.

I don't care what my blood tests say, I feel awful and need help.

Given my description of the physiology, it would make sense to expect a hormone test to tell you where you are in your menopause. Unfortunately, it is not as simple as that. Although the hormones show a predictable pattern during the pre-menopausal years and during post-menopause (remember: that is one year after periods stop), they go a bit wild around peri-menopause. It is during this time of peri-menopause that it would be most helpful to have a blood test that reliably confirms you are 'menopausal'. The two main hormones I mentioned, follicle stimulating hormone (FSH) and oestrogen, do change as you go through the menopause, but not in a smooth, predictable way. FSH rises as oestrogen levels fall, but you can have months when the hormones seem to be acting normally and others when they are very erratic. During this time you may be experiencing menopausal symptoms or you may not. You may miss some periods or you may not. The erratic changes can occur even over a few days, which means that the blood tests become very unreliable and may even give a false picture. You may go to your doctor with symptoms, which are apparently related to the menopause, but because the hormone levels don't conform to an expected pattern, you are told these symptoms don't need treatment. You still feel awful and leave the surgery confused and frustrated.

Guidance in the UK now tells clinicians that hormone tests are not needed to diagnose menopause or to start treatment for menopausal symptoms in women over the age of 45. Instead, the clinician listens to you and makes the diagnosis by building up a picture of how you might be approaching menopause, including what is happening to your periods and how you are feeling. Someone skilled in listening to menopausal women soon develops the expertise to recognise what is likely to be menopause. If there is any doubt, other medical tests might be done to rule out other medical causes for how you are feeling. These may include thyroid tests or iron levels. Most women, though, do not need any blood tests around the menopause. You may benefit from measurement of follicle stimulating hormone in the following situations:

- You are aged 40 to 45, so a little younger than average, and your symptoms and period pattern are not clearly menopausal, but you have symptoms suggesting it.
- You have a progestogen-releasing intrauterine system (coil or IUS) or progestogen-only pill contraception that has caused a lack of periods and now have symptoms and wonder if you are menopausal and can stop contraception (see Chapter 2).

◆ You are under 40 years of age and suspect menopause.

> ### Recommendation
> If you are under 40 years old and suspect menopause, it is essential to have at least two FSH tests, along with other health assessments as discussed in Chapter 5.

When hormone tests might not be accurate

FSH cannot be reliably measured if you are using the combined oral contraceptive pill ('the pill') or progestogen injection contraception (e.g. Depo). These forms of contraception suppress your natural hormonal cycle and any blood test will not reflect whether or not you are in menopause. FSH can be measured when using an IUS (e.g. Mirena or Jaydess), implant contraception (Nexplanon), or the progesterone-only pill, sometimes called the 'mini-pill'. On these types of contraception, your periods might have changed, perhaps stopping or becoming much lighter; this does not necessarily mean you are in menopause yet.

What are common symptoms?

Flushes and sweats

I wake three or four times a night, soaking wet and am constantly turning my pillow over to try and get cool.

At home, it's OK, we joke about it, but at work it is

embarrassing, and I try to cover it up. I leave the room sometimes, hoping no one will notice.

Flushes and sweats, or vasomotor symptoms, to give them their correct name, are probably the symptom that you will most identify as being due to menopause. If you see a stereotypical cartoon of a woman at menopause, she will undoubtedly be flushing or sweating. Many women experience these as they go through the peri-menopause and they often start before periods finally stop. In fact, if you miss a few periods these symptoms can worsen and then might improve again once you have another period, reflecting the changes in hormones during this transition. So you may have a few months when they are awful, then a few months when they subside, leading you to think they might be over, only for them to start all over again.

It is not clear exactly why some women get flushes and others don't or why sometimes they are severe and sometimes hardly a problem. Researchers are not even really sure why they happen around menopause so much, although there is a lot of research looking at genetic factors and other influences. Smoking may worsen flushes and you may notice that certain things trigger them off such as spicy foods, hot drinks, alcohol and feeling pressured for time. Even simply moving rooms from one temperature to another can set them off. Your internal 'thermostat' seems to function less efficiently making it harder to tolerate changes in temperature, without flushing or sweating.

They come from nowhere, the flushes, all of a sudden I start to feel strange then hot then I sweat …

I can feel it is about to start – I get an inner sense of it and think, Oh no, here it goes again.

Women describe these flushes as being a feeling of intense heat, that rises from within, commonly in the upper part of the body – the face, neck and shoulders in particular. Sometimes you go red in the face and sweat, but sometimes you don't. A flush may last a few moments or a few minutes. You may feel that your flush is visible to those around you, but often it is not and, even if it is, it may not be as noticeable as you think. At night, these flushes often turn into sweats, and you wake feeling first hot and then cold, clammy and uncomfortable. It might be so uncomfortable that you have to change sheets, nightclothes or even shower off to cool down. If you sleep with a partner, they may be disturbed and you both have a poor night's sleep, leaving you both tired and possibly grumpy in the morning. When this goes on night after night, month after month and sometimes year in year out, it is not surprising that women say that apparently minor symptoms like flushes can have a profound impact on quality of life.

How bad are they?

Flushes and sweats vary in intensity and will affect women in different ways. The severity of flushes are judged by how much they disturb you, so 'mild' flushes might not affect you very much at all: you are aware of them, but you carry on, and they only happen a couple of times a day or maybe once a night. You don't have to make adjustments and most people around you probably don't know they occur. 'Moderate' flushes might disturb you several times a day or night and may lead you to make changes such as changing to more comfortable work clothes, having fans around the bedroom or office, and finding ways to minimise the onset by looking at what triggers them or makes them worse. 'Severe' symptoms might occur several times an hour most days, and disturb you a few times each night. They may stop you living life to the full and impact on your ability to do your job or may limit your social activities. You might describe your flushes as moderate; someone else might consider them severe. It is how they affect you and the impact they have on your life that should determine whether you seek help, medical or otherwise. No clinician should tell you that your flushes 'are not bad enough' for treatment or that you should put up with them because they 'have seen worse'. You're the one who has to live with them.

Palpitations

The first time I felt my heart beating hard was scary; it was during a particularly bad sweat too.

After tests, my doctor reassured me there was nothing wrong with my heart. I was pleased, but I still had the palpitations and learnt to breathe myself through it.

This is when you get an awareness of your heart

pumping faster or harder than is usual. It can be unpleasant and you may worry that something is wrong with your heart. You may get palpitations during a hot flush or sweat or it may happen on its own as a symptom, often lasting just a few seconds or more. You may notice that it is worse after caffeine, cigarettes or alcohol, so limiting these can be beneficial. You may recognise these symptoms as part of an anxiety attack and dealing with underlying concerns may help resolve these symptoms too. Fortunately, these palpitations are not usually a sign of anything sinister, but it is worth getting them checked out to be sure.

Recommendation

If your irregular heartbeat is accompanied by dizziness or shortness of breath, always seek medical advice.

Tiredness

It is such an effort, I feel tired all the time and then at night, I just can't sleep, it is a never-ending cycle ...

I feel like an old lady – I get home from work and just collapse on the sofa.

As you go through the menopause, you might find yourself more tired than usual. This may be a direct consequence of not sleeping, particularly when the night sweats go on for months or even years. But poor sleep may not just be caused by disturbed nights; some women describe poor sleep as a menopause symptom itself, saying that it is difficult to get to sleep or they wake and then struggle to get back to sleep. You might wake for other reasons too such as needing to go to the loo, or with joint pains or another health-related condition. Stresses that often occur around the same time as menopause, like anxiety over work, family or relationships, will also interfere with good sleep and if you were never a particularly good sleeper, menopause just might make your insomnia worse. See Chapter 3 for tips on improving sleep at menopause.

Irregular periods

I had about four periods in the final year before they stopped altogether.

My periods became unpredictable, sometimes a month apart, sometimes three.

Often one of the first signs of menopause, a disruption to your cycle because of fluctuating hormones will inevitably result in irregular periods. It is unusual for periods to stop suddenly, although it does happen. It is much more likely that you will see a gradual change in period pattern, with them becoming further apart and there being an occasional missed period, until eventually they stop altogether. Before this happens, you may find that your periods get more frequent and sometimes more heavy in flow. This can cause anxiety and if your periods change a lot in pattern or flow, other than simply becoming less frequent, you should seek medical advice. The most common cause of irregular periods at this age is fluctuating hormone levels, but other factors may contribute, such as fibroids (non-cancerous growths), displaced coils, polyps and, very rarely, cancer.

Heavy menstrual bleeding is the term for excessive bleeding during a period. For example you might be bleeding for eight to ten days each month or passing clots on more than a couple of days. You may need to change pads or tampons every hour, may need to use both together and may get leakage onto your clothes. You may feel fatigued. Maybe you have flooding, which is when you have a sudden onset of a period that is very heavy. Your doctor will check for anaemia (low iron levels), will examine you, and may do an ultrasound scan to look for underlying causes. Your doctor may refer you for a hysteroscopy, which is a test using a fine telescope to look at the womb lining. Then treatment options can be discussed with you, which might be an intrauterine system (Mirena), medication or surgery.

Recommendation

See your doctor if your periods become much closer together, heavier than normal, you bleed for more than eight days each month or if you pass clots. If you go for a year without periods then have one, see your doctor.

Mood changes

I feel slightly out of control of my moods, and that worries me, it is just not normal for me to be like this.

I say and do things that are just not me; usually I am quite calm.

As if the physical symptoms aren't enough, you might also feel that your emotions have gone off balance. You feel fine one day then sad the next, in control one moment and then you lose it. Perhaps you are irritable, and sometimes you just feel plain angry. Mood swings during menopause are often related to the hormonal transitions that are occurring during this time. Hormones, such as oestrogen, influence the production of serotonin, which is a mood-regulating neurotransmitter. These changes can also contribute to symptoms like low mood. Coping with your daily physical menopausal symptoms might make you feel worn out, frustrated and anxious and, of course, the night-time disruption will not help your moods. Sometimes, your life experiences may increase the like-lihood of you having mood swings around menopause. If other times of hormonal change, like pregnancy or pre-period have been troublesome, menopause might be too, although it is never inevitable. Memories of past traumas or life events may rise within you again when you feel emotionally low at menopause; some women find counselling to be of benefit. Stress, such as illness, work issues or relationship difficulties, will also have an impact on your emotional health at this time. As you go through menopause, you may face a multitude of factors that will contribute to how well you feel; these may include:

◆ Care of ageing parents
◆ Adult children causing anxieties – leaving home or not leaving home!
◆ Relationship issues – partners, family members, work colleagues
◆ Attitude towards your own ageing and that of others around you
◆ Financial problems
◆ Loneliness or feeling isolated.

All of these can increase the likelihood of mood swings during menopause. If left unaddressed, you may see a negative effect on your personal relationships and at work. Understanding why they occur and acknowledging them is the first step towards achieving emotional balance. You can approach mood swings with lifestyle changes, therapy approaches and with medication. These are discussed in Chapter 3. HRT may have a role to play for some women and is discussed in Chapter 4.

My doctor kept blaming my hormones, but it is more than that; I think I might be depressed.

Clinical depression is different to low mood and although menopause can be a trigger for depression in susceptible women, it is rarely the sole cause. If you or those around you suspect that you might be depressed, seek help from your doctor or another health professional.

Bear in mind that it is possible to be depressed and menopausal: you may need treatment or support for both.

Recommendation

If you or those around you suspect depression, seek medical advice.

Irritability

I am usually quite calm, but I blow off the handle at the slightest thing.

I constantly feel 'on edge', keeping my temper in line.

You may find yourself less tolerant of others' weaknesses, quicker to snap and less able to rein in your anger, especially with those closest to you. Hormonal fluctuations around menopause influence mood and so do ongoing physical symptoms and tiredness. Knowing that it happens is important because then you can tackle it, perhaps by using techniques such as relaxation and deep breathing, by taking 'time out' from the moment, and by putting in place strategies to help you, such as minimising stress and pressures where possible. Try to build a personal support system around you of friends or family who can be honest but supportive. Simple changes to diet and exercise may also help, along with addressing those physical symptoms that might be contributing to your overall well-being. Sleep disturbance is a common cause of irritability so dealing with this issue alone may improve the situation.

Memory lapses

It's the small things I forget, where I put things, what I meant to buy on the way home …

It becomes a family joke that I forget things, but it is not funny when it is you, and it happens time and time again.

Both men and women have changes in memory over time and it is normal to have lists and reminders, as you get older, just to keep up with busy lives. Menopause, though, can worsen those lapses and make you feel bad because of it. Forgotten birthdays, lost keys and the like may lead to feelings of disappointment in yourself and can make you start feeling anxious. Some women describe it as 'brain-fog', and it can be similar to what you experienced in pregnancy, when hormones were also fluctuating widely. Changes in oestrogen during the menopause contribute to this, as does stress, poor sleep and putting pressure on yourself through overwork. You could try the following:

◆ Change the way you remember – don't just rely on verbal reminders, write things down.

◆ Use electronic reminders on your phone or computer – these then become both visual and timely.

◆ Keep your brain active through crosswords, sudoku and puzzles if your daily work does not do this.

◈ Physical exercise has been shown to help brain function – another reason to get on with it!

> ### Recommendation
>
> Occasional memory lapses are not usually signs of dementia, but if you or those around you are concerned, seek medical advice.

Joint pains (Arthralgia)

It's not really pain, just a real achy feeling in my joints.

I get up in the morning and feel like an old woman.

Joint pains are interesting because the relationship between this symptom and hormones is unclear and joint pains can be a sign of ageing, not just hormonal activity. Yet many women describe these around the time of the menopause and, interestingly, some report an improvement with the use of hormone replacement therapy.

Joints, commonly the wrists and knees but also the neck and shoulders, become sore, stiff and sometimes swollen. The discomfort may seem worse first thing in the morning and may be mild, occurring mainly when you are active, or more severe, limiting movement. It is worth getting joint pains checked out, especially if they are accompanied by:

◆ Swelling

◆ Redness

◆ Tenderness and warmth around the joint.

Skin changes and hair loss

I am in my forties. I thought only teenagers got acne.

My hair has changed; it used to be thick and glossy, now it's a bit thinner everywhere.

Menopause affects the outside of the body as well as the inside. Collagen production changes and the balancing of hormones can lead to greater testosterone effects such as oily skin, occasional facial hair and acne-type spots. Other skin changes are usually a combination of factors relating to ageing and hormones and may include:

◆ Dry skin

◆ Loss of elasticity, leading to wrinkles

◆ Itching or a strange sensation of crawling on the skin.

Partly because of ageing effects, menopausal skin is more susceptible to skin damage, so if you do not already use sun protection on your skin, now would be a good time to start. Hormones affect the production of melatonin, which is the body's way of adapting to sun exposure, and you may see an overproduction in some areas of previously exposed skin, for example your neck and arms. This can result in the brown patches, often unfairly called 'age spots'.

> **Recommendation**
>
> If you see a new area of pigmentation that is growing, or a mole that is changing in size or appearance, seek medical advice.

You may notice a general thinning of your hair, which is a gradual process and extends to body hair such as pubic hair. It is unusual to see patches of hair loss or baldness due only to menopause, so if this happens it is worth seeking medical advice. It may be that you have a vitamin deficiency or it may be a sign of another illness. It is normal to see some changes in hair at menopause, but hair also reflects general health, stress and anxiety as well as hormones.

Weight gain

It creeps on, suddenly your clothes are tight, and then you are looking at larger sizes.

I feel my waistline is thicker even though I weigh the same.

Is weight gain a menopausal symptom? There is no doubt that women often feel that they have gained weight because of menopause, yet many don't change weight. Between the ages of 45 and 55, many women will indeed gain weight but not always directly as a result of hormonal changes due to menopause; it may be that some women are more susceptible to weight gain at menopause in the same way that some women gain more in pregnancy than others. Certainly, as women age, there is a change in weight distribution across the body, with an increase around the middle area leading to the so-called 'middle-aged spread'. Metabolism also changes, meaning that you need to reduce food intake simply to maintain the same weight. So if you continue to eat what you did when younger then the weight will creep on. Losing weight around menopause is a challenge but can be done with a little know-how and a lot of support. See Chapter 2 for advice on managing weight.

You may find that going through menopause makes you rethink your lifestyle and eating habits and that you take up a healthier pattern of eating than you have done in the past. Preventing weight gain at menopause is about making positive dietary changes and maintaining or increasing exercise. Remember too that alcohol adds to calorie intake and can be a hidden contributing factor to weight gain.

Bladder symptoms

When you have to go, you really have to go!

I plan my trip around toilet stops. I just can't hold.

Bladder symptoms make you uncomfortable – in more ways than one. The actual symptoms are a nuisance and then talking about them is embarrassing. Do you really want to admit to having some leakage, or to feelings of urgency? It all feels somewhat unfeminine and brings home the issues of ageing. So you might avoid discussing it, invest in some of the pretty panty liners on the market and ignore it, or put up with it. You would be joining many other silent women in the same situation and this is a real shame because sometimes treatments for bladder symptoms are quite simple. Doctors are used to talking about it, so if this is a problem for you, ask for help.

Stress or Overactive Bladder (OAB) or both?

Bladder symptoms are defined for diagnostic purposes in one of two ways, and you may relate more to one than the other: stress incontinence or overactive bladder (OAB). You may have a mixture of both, which is also very common.

I have to wear pads at my exercise class, but otherwise I'm OK.

I only have to laugh aloud, or cough and I leak slightly.

Stress incontinence is when you leak urine as you cough, sneeze or exercise. It happens because the pelvic floor weakens with age and after having children. If you have scrupulously done your pelvic-floor exercises over the years, you may have kept the muscles strong and even now it is never too late to start them. Many women can significantly improve mild leakage by commencing and continuing pelvic-floor exercises. If you carry extra weight, losing some might also help your bladder symptoms. See Resources chapter for more information on how to do effective pelvic-floor exercises.

Overactive bladder (OAB)

Just as I put my key in the door, I have an urgency that I can't hold.

I go to the loo, then an hour later, I have to go again.

You might not get leakage with coughing at all; your problem might be urgency, not getting to the toilet in time, or having to go more frequently and then feeling as if you did not empty your bladder. You may be getting up several times a night and going more than around eight times a day. You might leak, or you might not quite get there in time. If this is you, do speak to your doctor, as help is available, often in the form of tablets and, if very troublesome, through bladder health clinics.

Infections

I went through a phase when I felt I had continual cystitis but urine samples kept coming back clear.

If you have bladder symptoms, the first step is to rule out urine infections, which are also very common around the time of the menopause. Symptoms of an infection include:

◆ Passing urine frequently
◆ Pain or feeling of burning on passing urine
◆ Urine that smells strongly and is cloudy
◆ Pain – Pelvic or abdominal.

A simple urine test can check for infection and identify which particular antibiotics will treat it. Sometimes, it can feel as if you have an infection but samples come back clear of bacteria. There is no point in taking repeated antibiotics in this instance; rather, your doctor should be looking at other ways to treat your bladder symptoms, which might include local vaginal oestrogen (see Chapter 4).

It is embarrassing to discuss this.

It is easier to buy pads than face going to the doctor.

Bladder symptoms seldom get better on their own accord. Your clinician should put you at ease in discussing these problems and should help you to find ways to improve them. It might seem a tricky topic but bladder symptoms can have a tremendous impact on your everyday life, so it is worth seeking help rather than just putting up with them.

Low sex drive

It feels like such an effort, I often just can't face it.

Many women say that they lose some of their sex drive as they go through menopause. Sex drive in women is complicated. Hormones play a vital role but so do other factors. Loss of sex drive, or libido, is described as a lack of interest in sexual activity. You may feel that the sexual feelings of the past have gone and that even the thought of sex is tiresome, too much hard work and not worth the effort. If the lack of interest in sex distresses you, note that the medical term used for it is 'female sexual interest/arousal disorder' – FSIAD. Lack of desire differs from lack of response and sometimes women will respond naturally once sex is initiated even though the desire may be slow in coming forward. There are physical and psychological aspects to this and it may help to look at each in turn.

Physical changes

The hormonal fluctuations around menopause include a gradual decline in testosterone, often wrongly described as a 'male hormone'. Women too have testosterone throughout life and changing testosterone levels may play a role in decreasing desire for sex. However, the answer is not always to simply replace testosterone because so many other factors contribute to positive sexual function and should, therefore, also be addressed. If poor sex drive continues once other aspects have been dealt with, some clinicians will consider a trial of testosterone therapy under careful supervision (see Chapter 4).

Vaginal dryness

Sex is painful, I want it, but now I am tense before we even start, as I am anxious it will hurt.

I feel my natural lubrication has gone awry.

The lack of oestrogen around peri-menopause and especially in the years after menopause means that the sexual organs are affected, the vagina in particular. You might notice itching, less natural lubrication, and that lovemaking is uncomfortable or painful. This is because the vaginal walls become thinner, less elastic, and lose tone after menopause and with age. Usually made up of plump, soft tissue, the vagina becomes a little less elastic and prone to bleeding. Some women will not notice the change, but for others this can result in 'vaginal atrophy', the medical term used to describe the physiological changes that can lead to symptoms such as vaginal dryness and painful sex. While some women experience vaginal symptoms at the time of peri-menopause, for many it does not become a problem until four to five years later and in the years beyond menopause. You may also experience an increase in the need to pass water and feel like you sometimes have a bladder infection, but there is no infection when tested. This combination of mild bladder symptoms and vaginal dryness, and the consequence of painful sex, are described as 'urogenital menopause symptoms'. Treatments are discussed in Chapters 3 and 4.

Body image

I look in the mirror and see an old woman – it's not me, surely?

Coming as it does naturally at midlife, the menopause can be a reminder that you are getting older. The end of your periods is tangible evidence that your child-bearing days are over. For some this may be a relief, for others it brings pain, even if you thought that you had come to terms with not having children. Society influences our attitudes, often leading us to believe that middle-aged women are invisible or unattractive. Attitudes around menopause can affect self-esteem, and negative self-image may contribute to a loss of sexual desire. Young women see reminders all around that menopause is associated with ageing, and it can be difficult for women experiencing early menopause to remember that many of the changes seen in middle-aged women at menopause are due to ageing and not just to hormones.

Talking about it to professionals

You may feel embarrassed about talking to your doctor about such intimate issues, but the treatment of vaginal symptoms is usually easy and once you start the discussion, treatments can be discussed. Sex is part of health and well-being and all health professionals should feel at ease discussing it and offering help as a natural part of their care. In order to promote discussion you could say:

- I have found that lovemaking is becoming uncomfortable: can you suggest something to help?
- Sex is more difficult, I may be dry – can you offer some treatment?
- I know menopause can lead to vaginal dryness – how can I address this?

Recommendation

If you get bleeding after sex, seek medical advice.

Talking about it to your partner

It is important to be open with your partner about your thoughts on sex before misunderstandings start to creep in. You may feel that your partner is being insensitive by still wanting to make love; they may feel rejected and unloved when you don't. You may inadvertently be closing down on your sexual relationship because you are keen to avoid potentially painful sex but actually be closing down on all intimacy simply because of poor communication. Each of you may be avoiding the conversation and arguments may result. Satisfaction within the relationship, emotional stability as a couple, and the psychological well-being of both partners all contribute to a healthy sex life. If a problem exists, it probably exists for you both although each of you may be affected in different ways. This is a time for patience and understanding on both sides. For tips about discussing sex and relationships, take a look at Relate – www.relate.org.uk. Details in the Resources section.

Other effects on your health

Menopausal symptoms are troublesome enough, but the lack of oestrogen caused by menopause will also impact on parts of the body that you might not consider to have anything to do with hormones, in particular, your heart and bones. This is particularly important for young women (see Chapter 5), but every woman should be aware that hormones and the loss of oestrogen after menopause have an impact on heart and bone health.

Bones

I thought osteoporosis only affected old women.

It wasn't until I broke a bone, that I even thought about my bones; I mean, they are just there, doing their job, aren't they?

Osteoporosis is a common condition and affects women more often than men. It occurs when bone density declines to such an extent that bones are more fragile and fracture more easily. It is slow to develop and silent; you are not aware of the changes until much later in life when fractures may occur.

Bone continues to grow throughout life. New bone develops and replaces bone that is naturally destroyed by activity at cellular level. You are unaware of this growth as it does not result in any changes that you can see and any damage to this process of bone reformation is silent, causing no pain until you get a fracture, often out of the blue and sometimes after only a slight fall or injury. Hormonal influences are crucial and up to the time of menopause, bone turnover in healthy women is fairly constant, causing no problems unless there are medical conditions that might affect bone turnover, for example rheumatoid arthritis.

After menopause, at whatever age that occurs, you experience a more rapid turnover in bone, to the extent that it cannot keep up with the rate of bone loss and you start to see a decline in bone density or strength. Both men and women lose bone density with age, but women have this additional hormone-related bone loss around menopause. This accelerated bone loss may last up to ten years after menopause and eventually will go back to the steady rate of loss associated with ageing. In some women, the bone loss will be sufficient to cause bone thinning, which could lead to an increased risk of fracture. This is called osteopenia, the stage before osteoporosis. You will be unaware of the deterioration, but there are some warning signs (or risk factors) that you should be aware of:

- Previous fracture – if you break your wrist following a relatively minor fall, for example tripping on the pavement, that could be an early warning sign that your bones are thinning.

- Low body mass index – if you are petite in build and thin, you have a greater risk of developing osteoporosis.

- Family history – if either of your parents had signs of osteoporosis, such as a fractured hip or curvature of the spine, you might be more likely to get it too.

- Medications – certain medications, such as steroid treatment, thyroid therapy and anti-epileptic medicines, can affect your bone health, sometimes speeding up the bone loss that leads to osteoporosis. You should not stop the treatment without medical advice, but your doctor may advise monitoring bone density around the time of menopause if you use these medicines.

- Smoking – as well as being bad for other aspects of your health, smoking is bad for bones: yet another reason to quit.

◆ Alcohol – heavy alcohol drinking has a harmful effect on bone health and can increase the risk of falling.

◆ Early menopause – menopause before the age of 40 leads to the early onset of accelerated bone loss, which HRT will prevent. If someone has had long stretches of time without periods for other reasons, e.g., anorexia or over-exercising, this will also affect bones.

How will you know if you are at risk of osteoporosis?

After my wrist fracture, I had a DXA and that told me I had osteoporosis.

All women are at risk, with some having a higher risk than others. Look at the risk factors above and seriously review whether you fit some of the higher risk groups. If you do, discuss with your doctor whether it would be useful to have a measurement of bone density performed. This simple test (called DEXA or DXA) uses X-Ray to measure segments of your skeleton in order to assess risk for osteoporosis. It is non-invasive: you simply lie on a couch and the machine does the rest – no tunnels or tubes. DEXA measures your bone density at the hip and the spine, areas that are known to be indicative of skeletal health generally. If you want to assess your personal risk further and don't mind using online calculation tools, the FRAX tool (https://www.shef.ac.uk/FRAX/tool.jsp) enables you to assess personal risk of fracture. You enter in various details about yourself, and it offers a prediction of ten-year risk of fracture. You can use this information to discuss with your doctor whether a bone scan might be useful. You will find more information about this in in the Resources section and in Chapter 2, which also covers steps you can take to minimise bone loss, including dietary changes, exercise and lifestyle changes.

Heart

You may think that heart disease prevention messages are for men. The stereotypical heart attack occurs in a middle-aged, overweight and overworked man, yet women too can get heart disease and symptoms in women may be different to those in men. Heart disease affects more women every year than breast cancer, yet heart disease is still considered by many to be 'a man's disease'. Why is this? It is partly because men seem to get their heart attacks sooner than women. You may not realise that female hormones play a protective role in the heart until menopause occurs so if menopause occurs early, the risk of heart disease starts earlier too. After the menopause, women 'catch up' with men and, as a woman, you need to be as aware of your heart health as you are of your breast health.

At around the age of 40, the NHS sometimes offers a health check for heart disease. These tests will help identify anything that might indicate a higher personal risk, e.g. high blood pressure or high cholesterol. A family history of heart disease is relevant too, and you should seek advice if:

- Your father or brother was under the age of 55 when they were diagnosed with cardiovascular disease; or

- Your mother or sister was under the age of 65 when they were diagnosed with cardiovascular disease.

As with your bones, certain factors will indicate a higher risk for heart disease. Some of these you cannot change, like family history or your age, but others you can influence:

- Smoking – increases the risk of heart disease and stroke by a factor of two to four, and for women, smoking is thought to be even more harmful to the heart than it is for men.

- Weight – being overweight puts a strain on your heart, raises blood pressure and cholesterol and increases your risk of diabetes.

- Blood pressure – high blood pressure makes your heart work harder and if untreated can lead to long-term damage.

- Lack of physical activity – a sedentary lifestyle increases the risk of high blood pressure and heart attacks.

- High cholesterol – over time, cholesterol hardens into plaque and causes narrowing of the arteries, reducing circulation and increasing risk of clots.

> **Recommendation**
>
> Symptoms you should never ignore:
>
> ◆ Frequent palpitations
> ◆ Shortness of breath
> ◆ Pressure feelings in the chest
> ◆ Lightheadedness and dizziness.

It is never too late to take steps to prevent heart disease. In Chapter 2 there is information about how you can look after your heart health through lifestyle, diet, exercise and, if appropriate, medication.

Are you under 40 years old?

I am only 30: does all this apply to me?

If you are young when you go through menopause, your experience will be different. Your symptoms may present differently and the health implications of menopause become more significant. You will be dealing with the physical changes and the psychological implications of early menopause. If you are supported through both aspects, you will emerge positive and in good health from both a hormonal point of view and a psychosocial one. Yes, you will have to make adjustments, and you will have to consider the long-term health effects of early menopause, such as osteoporosis prevention and heart health, making menopause management a crucial topic for you. You may need extra emotional support, too, as you come to understand the diagnosis and all its implications. See Chapter 5 for more information.

It is not all negative

At last I have seen the end of PMT.

Menopause just came and went – no big deal.

It is just another passage of life we have to go through.

So is there such a thing as 'normal menopause'? Most women will get some symptoms, some worse than others. Most women will acknowledge the symptoms, cope with them, and look forward to them ending. Thankfully, very few women get an abundance of symptoms, and some women get none at all. For you, menopause might simply be a passage of time over which your periods stop, with few symptoms and with no need to seek help. This too is normal.

The impact of the symptoms will vary according to the demands of your life, the support you have around you and the nature of your symptoms. Whether or not you seek medical help will be dictated very much by your attitude towards medication and how bothersome you find the symptoms. For most women, treating menopausal symptoms is a choice, and only you can weigh up if it is necessary.

Menopause may be a challenge for some but it does not have to be. Our bodies let us know that changes are occurring, some more dramatic than others, but we can't blame everything that happens on hormones. Life itself throws us challenges and the way we cope or respond to these will depend largely on our character, strengths, and supportive relationships, not just on our hormones. When menopause occurs at the usual time, you may see menopause as an end, a negative experience. For others, it is a beginning – the start of a new phase of life, where priorities change and life takes on a new pattern. This is as much about ageing as it is about menopause, and about how society puts an emphasis on staying youthful. How you regard ageing will be influenced by your satisfaction with life, your relationships and your work, as well as how you experience the physical changes of menopause.

Top tips for a positive menopause

- Know your options – it is your decision how you live through menopause, and your choices may be different to that of others.
- Develop techniques to cope with negative thinking about ageing and menopause.
- Explore treatment options for troublesome symptoms if you have them and seek help when needed.
- Be informed – about health consequences and symptoms.
- Make positive lifestyle changes to improve health (see Chapter 2).
- Don't confuse menopause with stress or ageing. The reality is that the way you feel can be a consequence

of all three. Address those that you can and accept what cannot be changed.

Reasons to look forward to natural menopause

◆ No more periods.

◆ PMS is a thing of the past.

◆ Cyclical bloating is over, along with the breast soreness before every period.

◆ You can forget contraception (eventually!).

◆ It can be a time for you to re-evaluate your health and make positive changes for the future.

◆ It is a time of choice – manage it your way.

◆ Enjoy the wisdom that comes with age.

◆ Menopause may mark the beginning of new chapters in life – plan for them and enjoy.

Frequently asked questions

1 *How do I know I am in menopause?*

If you are around the usual age of menopause, your body will start to let you know that menopause might be soon. You are likely to get symptoms as well as changes in relation to your periods, either of which may be the first sign that hormones are changing and that menopause is on its way. Sometimes periods change first, sometimes the symptoms come first – either is normal.

2 *What if I am much younger, how will I know this is menopause?*

If you are under the age of 40, your first warning signs might be a change in periods, perhaps getting much lighter or further apart. You may get symptoms, or you may not. A numbers of conditions can lead to missed periods so if you miss periods for more than three months, or have more than six months of irregular periods, get checked out.

3 *Isn't menopause natural, so why should I consider HRT?*

Menopause that occurs after the age of 45 is natural and you may not need HRT. If your symptoms are particularly bothersome, making life difficult or work hard, you may decide that you need help and support in order to cope with them. This might include HRT. If you are younger, menopause may not be considered 'natural' and you will be offered the opportunity to discuss HRT for long-term health benefits (see Chapter 5).

4 *How long do symptoms last?*

This is very individual. Many women will see symptoms for a couple of years or so, quite a few for around four to five years and a few women will see them last for many years, into their sixties and beyond. Some women will see very few symptoms at all and changes in periods will be the only outward sign of menopause.

5 *Should I see a doctor when I go through menopause?*

Some women choose to see a clinician to discuss how to manage troublesome symptoms. Others review their personal health and consult a health professional to discuss how to minimise risk for future illness, perhaps at the NHS Health Check or at another time. This will depend on your personal and family medical history (see Chapter 2). Many women will not consult a health professional at this time as they feel that there is no need; the choice is yours.

6 *How do I know if a particular symptom is due to menopause, or to something else like stress?*

Sometimes you will not know and many symptoms will be worsened by multiple factors. Menopausal symptoms often come in 'clusters' so you may get a few symptoms, which together appear to suggest that they may be due to menopause. You may also get 'domino' symptoms, when you experience direct consequences of a symptom, which leads to other symptoms. For example, if night sweats keep you awake night after night, you may feel tired and irritable. If you are able to deal with the night sweats, the tiredness and irritability might go too – an added benefit of treating just one symptom.

7 *What causes women to have menopause?*

Usually the menopause is a natural consequence of the ovaries ageing. In some women, menopause may be caused by cancer treatments or by medical conditions that affect the healthy ovary, and sometimes ovaries stop working in young women for no known reason.

8 *Should I treat menopause?*

Whether or not you decide to treat your menopause will depend on many factors. How bothersome are your symptoms? What would you gain by using a medical treatment (HRT) and, for you, what might any risks or side effects be? Can you manage without HRT? A few women are advised to use HRT for health reasons; most have a choice. That is why you need reliable information – to make an informed decision that is right for you.

9 *My mother had an early menopause; should I be worried?*

There could be a variety of reasons for your mother's early menopause. Early menopause can sometimes run in families so if there was no obvious cause for it, then there may be a genetic factor in the family. It is by no means conclusive though, so if you are concerned, discuss it with your doctor.

10 *My mother had a terrible time with the menopause – does that mean I will?*

There is no evidence that we follow the pattern of our mothers in terms of severity of menopausal symptoms or how long they last. Your menopause experience will be unique to you.

11 *My friends seem very bothered by symptoms, but I don't get any. Is this normal?*

You may just be one of the small number of women who don't notice any symptoms as they go through menopause – be pleased! If you have not yet seen a change in periods, you just might not have got there yet.

12 *I can't say I get a specific flush or sweat, but I am warm most of the time. Others comment on it. Could this be due to menopause?*

This may be the way that your body is changing to internal temperature controls – yes. Not every woman experiences classic flushes or sweats. For some, it's a more general rise in feelings of heat, occasionally associated with other symptoms like those discussed on pages 14–25.

13 *I have always enjoyed sex and am worried menopause will spoil this – is it inevitable that sex life deteriorates after menopause?*

Not at all. Menopause is just one factor to influence sex drive (see Chapter 2) and although you may need to address issues like vaginal dryness, you can still maintain a healthy sexual relationship. With communication and occasionally a little help from lubricants or vaginal oestrogen, your sex life can continue to be enjoyable in the years beyond menopause.

14 *My partner and I have stopped having sex. The relationship is fine, we just don't seem to need it any more. Is this abnormal?*

There is nothing to be concerned about if you are both happy with this. Assuming there is no conflict between you around sex, you are probably expressing intimacy and closeness in other ways.

15 *I had a hysterectomy, with my ovaries left behind, at the age of 42. I am now 47 and have flushes and sweats. Is this menopause? How do I know?*

This probably is menopause and because you do not have periods, you have lost the 'marker' that usually tells you that it's starting. Flushes and sweats are classic menopausal symptoms and you are of usual menopause age (if on the young side of average), so yes, it is probably menopause. Unless you have other less classic symptoms, you can assume this is menopause and make your choices as to how to deal with them.

The next chapter will consider ways of looking after your health around menopause and discuss ways of making lifestyle changes that will promote good health not just around the menopause but also into the years ahead. Subsequent chapters look at treatment options and at specific groups of women for whom menopause might be just a bit more challenging.

chapter 2

Staying healthy through menopause

Positive lifestyle changes that will make a difference

Fab after fifty: that's what they say, isn't it!

If you reflect on how menopause is portrayed in women's magazines and social media, you will notice that the message is often about getting through menopause while staying young-looking and sexy, and of course going through the symptoms as best you can. Where is the recognition that menopause, at the usual time, is natural, inevitable and simply part of life? What about the positives, the freedoms, the maturity and the life experience? Looking after your health at menopause includes reviewing not just your physical well-being, but also your emotional, psychological and, for some, spiritual health. HRT is not the answer to all these, and you will want to look much more holistically at ways of improving health in all areas of your life as you go through the transition of menopause.

Menopause usually occurs around midlife and in this chapter I will outline some areas of your health where making positive changes at this time will benefit you, not just now but for the future – life beyond menopause and into the years ahead. If you are young, you may see things differently and have different priorities, but the advice will be similar for you too – incorporating into your life those elements of a healthy lifestyle that promote health, not hinder it. The key areas are:

◆ Heart health
◆ Bone health
◆ Stress management
◆ Healthy eating
◆ Sexual health (including contraception)
◆ Health screening.

Menopause may occur at any age, and if you go through menopause at a young age, under 40, you will be recommended hormone replacement in order to keep healthy and to prevent the onset of conditions like osteoporosis and heart disease. If you go through menopause at the usual age of around 50, you may not need HRT but you will still want to stay healthy through the menopause and into the years beyond. Menopause is natural and you cannot prevent it even if you want to. The chance of developing some illnesses, however, increases after menopause, and there are steps you can take to improve how you feel, lower the risks of age-related diseases, and live longer healthily. With natural menopause occurring around midlife, it is an excellent opportunity to look at how you live, make positive changes for the future, and invest in good health. It may be some time before you reap the benefits, but you will be pleased that you did.

Menopause and the heart

You may not think of heart disease as a female issue and you may worry more about diseases like breast cancer or dementia. Coronary heart disease is the most common cause of death for women over the age of 50 and is thought to kill at least twice as many women as breast cancer. Heart disease often occurs later in life in women than it does in men and the menopause is significant because, before it, the risk of a heart attack in women is low. After menopause, the risk rises and continues to increase as you get older. The good news is that you can take steps to reduce the risk of heart disease after menopause.

Coronary heart disease begins when your arteries start to become blocked with a gradual build up of fatty material, which at first causes no problems. Over the years this increases to such an extent that if the arteries become very blocked, oxygen to your heart is restricted and you get pain, called angina. Angina may be worse with exercise or triggered by being emotionally upset. If the artery becomes completely blocked, you may have permanent damage to the heart and have a heart attack or myocardial infarction. You may think that men mainly get heart attacks, but women too can get them.

Recognising your risk

The British Heart Foundation highlights risk factors for heart disease. That means that these may increase your chance of developing heart disease if they apply to you:

◆ Smoking

◆ High blood pressure

◆ High cholesterol

◆ Physically inactive

◆ Being overweight or obese

◆ Diabetes

◆ A family history of heart disease at a young age (under 55 for men and under 65 for women)

◆ Age (higher risk as you get older)

◆ Ethnic background: If you are from a South Asian or black African background, you are at a higher risk of CHD and stroke. Some risk factors appear to have a greater effect on this group of people. For example, those from South Asian backgrounds tend to put on weight around their middle, increasing their risk of CHD, stroke and diabetes.

You cannot change all these risk factors, for example your age, your family history or ethnic background, but there is plenty you can do through healthy lifestyle choices to lessen the risk of heart disease. Given that it is the accumulation of risk factors that is important, even changing some of these could have a positive impact on your future health.

Smoking

> One in five women in the UK smoke. Women who smoke have nearly twice the risk of having a heart attack, compared with women who have never smoked.
>
> *Women and heart disease*, British Heart Foundation Publication, 1 October 2013

Everyone accepts that smoking is bad for your health, even smokers. Stopping smoking is probably the single most beneficial step you can take to improving health, and within one year of quitting you will have reduced your risk of heart disease by half. Stopping smoking is not easy and getting support through it is vital. Ask about a local smoking cessation service at your surgery or pharmacy or see the Resources section of this book for organisations that can help you quit. As well as benefiting your heart, other reasons to stop smoking include:

◆ Better for your bone health
◆ Improve your lung function and lessen risk of lung disease
◆ Improve skin and teeth, including your breath
◆ Smoking may worsen flushes and sweats
◆ Sense of taste will return
◆ Save money!

Blood pressure

About 30 per cent of women in the UK have high blood pressure.

Women and heart disease, British Heart Foundation Publication, 1 October 2013

High blood pressure is sometimes described as a silent threat because it does not usually cause any symptoms: you will not know it is high unless you have it checked. Having a high blood pressure significantly increases your risk of a heart attack or stroke, so if it is found to be persistently high, your doctor will suggest medication to reduce it.

I bought myself a machine, but I had no idea what the numbers meant!

Blood pressure is expressed as two figures, usually given as one number over another number, for example, 130 over 80, or 130/80. If your blood pressure is consistently above 140/90, it is considered to be high. If you have a single high reading, you will need to have it checked and might be asked to record your blood pressure for a couple of weeks at home.

It's not always clear what causes high blood pressure, but certain things can increase the chances of it:

◆ Age – blood pressure rises with age
◆ Being overweight
◆ If you are of African or Caribbean descent
◆ Having a relative with high blood pressure, e.g. parent or sibling

◆ Having a diet rich in salt and not enough fruit and vegetables

◆ Not taking enough exercise

◆ Drinking too much alcohol or coffee (or other caffeine-based drinks)

◆ Smoking

◆ Not getting much sleep or having disturbed sleep.

Making healthy lifestyle changes will help reduce your chances of developing high blood pressure and help lower it if it's already high. This includes:

◆ Reducing your salt intake and having a healthy diet

◆ Cutting back on alcohol, limiting to no more than fourteen units a week and having at least two days without alcohol a week

◆ Maintaining a healthy body weight

◆ Taking regular exercise (see section on exercise)

◆ Cutting down on caffeine

◆ Stopping smoking.

You can check blood pressure at your surgery and some pharmacies and it will be checked if you attend the NHS Health Check offered to most people between the ages of 40 and 74 in England. This health check aims to spot any signs of heart disease, diabetes, stroke and dementia early on and will help you to put in place strategies to minimise this risk. Such strategies will include making lifestyle changes and, if necessary, medication.

Alcohol

I thought a little alcohol was good for you?

Is alcohol good or bad for your heart? It all depends on how much of it you drink. A small amount might be beneficial, although not enough to take up drinking if you do not already do so. There are other more useful things you can do, like increasing exercise and keeping to a healthy weight.

Drinking alcohol to excess is not good for your heart and may be harmful. You should drink no more than around one to two units of alcohol a day, and then not every day. More than fourteen units a week will be more harmful and binge drinking your allowance all in one day is not a good idea either.

To give you some idea, here are some estimations of units in typical drinks (from Drinkaware):

◆ Average bottle of wine – 10 units
◆ Large glass wine (250ml) – 3.5 units
◆ Pint of higher-strength beer or lager – 3 units
◆ Bottle (330ml) lager – 1.7 units
◆ Pub measure of spirit (25ml) – 1 unit.

Tips for being alcohol-aware:

◆ Track your units – you could use charts, apps or diaries. At first, you might be surprised at how it adds up.
◆ Use a measure at home – be accurate, rather than overestimating. Home-poured drinks tend to be more generous than pub measures.

◆ Choose your times – when do you commonly drink? At dinner, in the evening or when out? Make choices that suit you.

◆ Aim for alcohol-free days each week – at least two.

Healthy eating for your heart

Eating a healthy balanced diet will help protect your heart as this will provide all the vitamins and nutrients you need. Healthy eating means:

◆ Five a day – at least five portions of fruit and vegetables each day.

◆ Choosing low-fat milk and dairy products.

◆ Eating less saturated fats – found in biscuits, cakes, pastries, pies. You do not have to avoid butter and oil completely but limit yourself to small amounts.

◆ Reducing sugar – watch out for 'ready meals' and convenience food, which are often high in sugar. Be aware that fruit juice and 'smoothies', while healthy, will add to your sugar intake.

◆ Lowering salt intake – watch out for ready-made sauces and meals and processed meats.

◆ Eating more fish – aim for at least two portions of oily fish a week, e.g. tuna, salmon, mackerel.

◆ Portion control – think about portion sizes when serving food: it is so easy to be generous.

Maintaining a healthy weight

The weight has crept on since menopause – I didn't even notice it.

It is not inevitable to gain weight at menopause, but many women say that maintaining their weight is a losing battle. A combination of a busy life, less time to exercise, a slower metabolism, and the consequences of ageing all change your body shape and can lead to weight gain.

A balanced, healthy diet will help maintain a healthy weight through menopause, which will reduce your risk of some diseases later in life, such as Type 2 diabetes, certain cancers, heart disease and stroke. Combined with exercise, you can work to lose weight; losing weight is hard work at any time and, it seems, especially so around menopause. It is natural to gain weight as you age, and if you do not reduce your total calorie intake, compared to when you were younger, or if you slow down on the exercise, it will creep on. Weight gain is not inevitable, but it takes intention, determination and, if possible, kindly support from others to prevent it. The menopause itself may contribute to weight gain, as metabolism changes, often slowing down. You may feel that your weight distribution changes slightly too, onto the middle or abdominal area, so-called 'middle-aged spread'. This affects some women more than others, and your genetic make-up will influence this as well as hormonal fluctuations.

Losing weight after the menopause works on the same principle as before – you need to take less in calories than you burn. Your metabolism will be lower than when you are younger, so you will not see the fast weight loss of your youth. Many weight loss diets will be successful; the secret is to find the one that fits with your life and that you can stick to. 'Quick fix' diets may help you lose weight in the short term, but unless you change the habits of a lifetime, it will go back on when you try to eat normally. Consider enlisting the support of a friend for mutual encouragement in weight loss. It may be that groups or online support will offer you the motivation and understanding to keep going when weight loss is slow, as it often is around menopause.

Some dietary changes to help lose weight might include:

1. Cut back on portion size.
2. Avoid soft drinks – stick to water when you can.
3. Minimise saturated fats – cakes, pastries, fried foods.
4. Focus on fruit and vegetables and use plenty to feel full.
5. Switch to wholegrain carbohydrates, unrefined grains that haven't had their bran and germ removed by milling, e.g. wholewheat pasta, brown rice, oats.

Increasing exercise while making dietary changes will help with weight control. If you are aiming to lose weight, it helps to aim for thirty minutes of aerobic exercise daily, such as walking, jogging, swimming or cycling. This is not always easy to achieve in a busy life or if you experience symptoms like tiredness and lack of energy.

Exercise

> Less than a third of women in England do enough physical activity to protect their heart.

British Heart Foundation physical activity statistics

Staying active is one way of lessening your risk of heart disease. Exercise will improve your cholesterol level, control weight and help to reduce stress. There are two main types of exercise that you need: cardiovascular and strength training.

Cardiovascular

Your heart needs daily exercise, to the extent that you feel warmer, get a little out of breath and make your heart beat faster. It should not be so hard that you cannot hold a conversation. The recommendation from the British Heart Foundation is for 150 minutes of activity a week, spread over the week. You could achieve this through walking briskly, joining a class such as Zumba, or taking up a forgotten sport like netball, hockey or tennis. Walking, dancing, cycling and swimming are all good for heart health, and even if you start with short periods of exercise that is still beneficial and may help you to build up to the recommended amount.

Strength training

In addition to cardiovascular exercise, you need activities at least twice a week that strengthen muscles. This might include exercising with weights or carrying heavy loads, like shopping bags or even gardening. If you join a gym, they will encourage you to add both strength and cardiovascular exercises into your exercise regimen.

Tips for building exercise into your life:

◆ Decide to exercise because you want to, not because you should – then you will find it easier to make time for it and might even enjoy it!

◆ Accept time constraints, 10–15 minutes activity is better than aiming for 30 minutes and failing. No guilt over missed exercise.

◆ Schedule your exercise – don't squeeze it out of your busy day.

◆ Join a friend – mutual support can be very encouraging, more fun and sociable too.

Recommendation

1. If you have a medical condition, seek the advice of your doctor before starting an exercise programme.
2. If exercise makes you feel dizzy, unwell or very breathless, ease up and see your GP.

Other benefits of regular exercise include:

◆ Helping to maintain healthy bone

◆ Increasing your metabolism and helping to maintain weight control

◆ Improving skin condition and elasticity

◆ Improving sleep and mood
◆ Reducing risk of some diseases, such as cancer, diabetes.

Menopause and bones

I thought only old women got osteoporosis; being told my bones are thin, at just 50 years, was a shock.

Throughout childhood and into young adulthood your bones are growing in strength until you reach your 'peak bone mass', the point at which your bones have developed in density as much as they ever will. Your individual peak bone mass will be influenced by your childhood activity levels, your diet and your hormones but also your genetic make-up, which you cannot change. Bone loss with age is natural, with some people losing bone faster than others, but there are ways it can be slowed down, thus reducing the risk of osteoporosis later in life. After the menopause, at whatever age it happens, you experience a period of faster bone loss. So menopause is seen as an important moment at which to look after the health of your bones and to try to minimise the impact of bone loss by improving those factors that we do have some influence over, such as diet and exercise; and, if necessary, starting HRT. Improved bone health will mean a lesser risk of fractures, which can be painful and debilitating, later in life.

Having the menopause earlier than usual is one risk factor for thinning bones. Others include:

- Long-term use of steroid medicines (not inhalers)
- Family history, e.g. mother or father with a hip fracture, or loss of height
- Having a low body mass index; that is, being quite underweight (body mass index under 19)
- Drinking more alcohol than is recommended
- Smoking
- Some medical conditions, like those leading to poor gastric absorption (e.g. Crohn's), some inflammatory conditions and thyroid disease
- Having months without natural periods when a young adult, perhaps as a result of over-dieting, over-exercising or a hormonal disorder
- Some medicines that affect hormones, for example, used to treat breast cancer.

Risk assessment

Finding out that I am at risk of osteoporosis has empowered me to start weight-bearing exercise and look after my bones.

Identifying if you may be at risk of a condition is called 'risk assessment' and may involve your doctor doing tests or simply looking at your family history. For osteo-porosis, you may be considered at risk if you have one or more of the factors listed above and your doctor might make an assessment using an online tool like FRAX (see the Resources section). This helps to decide if further tests, such as a bone density measurement, are needed.

Bone density measurement (DEXA scan)

I was worried about having the DEXA but I need not have been; it was totally painless and quick and no tunnels involved.

Bone density is measured using Dual Energy X-Ray Absorptiometry (DEXA, or DXA), a very low level of radiation. Your result is compared to a healthy young woman and calculated to give a score (T-Score) against the average. Then your result is expressed like this:

◆ If your T-Score is -1 below or +1 above 0 (average), you are described as having normal bone density.

◆ If your T-Score is between -1 and -2.5, this is described as 'low bone mass' or sometimes 'osteopenia'.

◆ If your T-Score is less than -2.5, you are said to have osteoporosis.

It is important to remember that low bone mass itself is simply a marker of risk; it does not mean that fractures are inevitable. Whether or not you are offered treatment will depend on your age, your other risk factors, and other medical conditions, as well as whether or not you have already broken any bones. If you are taking HRT already, then you are already protecting your bones from further thinning for as long as you stay on it.

Healthy eating for bones

As well as the balanced diet that you need for your heart health, your bones also need extra nutrients in the form of calcium and vitamin D.

Calcium

Calcium is essential for bone health and you can usually get enough through diet. You need around 700 mg/day (some would say 1000 mg after menopause and more if you have osteoporosis: ask your doctor if this is you). The simplest way to get calcium is through dairy products like milk, cheese and yoghurts. If you avoid dairy, you can get calcium in foods such as broccoli, cabbage, tofu, soy drinks fortified with calcium, nuts, and fish where you eat the bones, such as sardines. See the Resources section for more information about sources of calcium.

Examples of calcium in foods

Semi-skimmed milk	200 ml	240 mg
Full-fat milk	200 ml	236 mg
Almond milk	200 ml	90 mg
Cheese such as cheddar	30 g	240 mg
Broccoli	120 g	112 mg
Almonds	30 g	75 mg
Yoghurt	125 ml	200 mg
Sardines	100 g	410 mg
Sesame seeds	one tablespoon	160 mg

Recommendation

If you choose calcium supplements, don't take too much: 1000 mg or less a day is unlikely to cause harm. Be aware of the additional calcium you are taking through diet.

Vitamin D

Vitamin D is essential for bone health and some is found in foods such as oily fish, eggs, red meat, and some fortified foods like cereals. In addition, you get vitamin D when it is made in reaction to the sunlight. Even in the UK, from March to September, you can usually get enough exposure outside as long as your arms or legs are uncovered for some of the day. This does not mean risking skin cancer by avoiding sunscreen but rather moderating its use, so that for at least part of the day you allow sunlight to reach your skin without allowing redness and burning.

You might want to consider vitamin D supplements of 10 mcg/day if:

1. You are indoors most of the time, even in summer.
2. You usually wear clothes that cover most of your skin when outside.
3. You have naturally dark skin, which may not make as much vitamin D as lighter skin.

Between October and March, everyone should consider using a vitamin D supplement in the UK, as the sunlight is not always sufficient to keep natural levels adequate. The government recommendation is that everyone considers 10 mcg a day during this time.

Exercise for bone health

If you are doing the types of exercise suggested for heart health, you are already protecting your bones too as any exercise will benefit bone. The only difference is that you need to ensure that you build weight-bearing exercise into your programme. Weight-bearing exercises are those that you do from standing, such as walking, dancing or jogging. In addition, the strengthening exercises discussed above will be of great benefit to bones. Exercise such as Pilates and yoga will help balance and suppleness. If you have osteoporosis, tell your instructor so she can advise if you should avoid any of the specific exercise positions.

Stress management

My flushes are worse when I put myself under pressure.

I need to allow more time, both mentally and physically, or I get anxious.

Stress can arise from anywhere – your home, your work and your environment. Your symptoms might cause you stress and then life events may lead to more stress. At menopause, a whole combination of factors might come together, sometimes leaving you feeling that you can't cope well or that life is stressful. Many of the stresses at menopause are life-related rather than hormone-related – children leaving home (or not leaving home), caring for elderly parents, holding down a busy job. For younger women the stresses might be different – finding the right treatment, talking about fertility, coming to terms with the diagnosis. In either case, learning to acknowledge stress and handle it in a way that is right for you will help to reduce anxiety and enable you to cope.

Tips for dealing with stress:

◆ Identify places and times that you feel stress. Avoid them or seek support in them.

◆ Find activities that help you 'switch off': this might be relaxation, exercise or listening to music. Build in relaxing time.

◆ Set realistic goals. Don't put unfair expectations on yourself – it is so easy to do this.

◆ Be politely assertive – learn to say no when necessary and admit when you need help.

◆ Talk about problems if you can, explain how you feel to others you trust, even if you are not looking for solutions. A good listener can really help.

Pressure is not all negative: it can motivate you to get a job done, to change something, or to address an ongoing issue. Pressure might build up to stress. You will deal with stress in your own particular way, and it is when you realise that your ways of coping are not working, that you feel anxious or even ill, that you might need to make changes. Try to recognise this in yourself and take steps to minimise stress.

Sexual health

No more contraception, no more periods? Sex is fun again.

Sex? I would prefer to curl up with a good book …

Sexual health is individual and your sex life after menopause will probably mirror what it was like before.

If you had an active sex life before menopause, then you should be able to continue. You may notice that it takes a little longer to become aroused and that your body is not so sensitive to touch, and this may lead to less interest in sex. You may feel that your sexual response is duller than it used to be. Lubrication will be less and good lubrication lends itself to good response. Changes in your body, such as gaining weight, vaginal dryness and other effects of ageing and menopause, may make you feel less sexy, which can also inhibit lovemaking. On the other hand, your home might be emptier, your time your own again, and sex might become more relaxing and enjoyable.

If you have vaginal dryness, a consequence of menopause, lovemaking might be uncomfortable or even painful. You can address this easily with lubricants, moisturisers or vaginal oestrogen (discussed in chapters 3 and 4). Many women are embarrassed to mention this to their partner, but communication is essential; you may be avoiding sex because it is painful, but your partner may think that you are avoiding intimacy for other reasons. Unless you discuss this you run the risk of misunderstandings creeping into the relationship. Consider how you want to display intimacy and bring sex back into your relationship while taking practical steps to prevent further pain.

Low desire

Sexual desire or libido declines naturally with age but for some women, they notice a real shift around the time of menopause. You do not feel as 'turned on' or 'in the mood' any more. This can lead to friction in relationships and frustration in both partners, and if not discussed can lead to isolation within a partnership – a sure-fire way to inhibit more lovemaking. Avoiding sex altogether may feel like an option but is unlikely to bring long-term harmony to a healthy relationship.

Hormones partly influence libido and the hormonal fluctuations of oestrogen and testosterone around the time of the menopause will play a part in lessening desire, more in some women than in others. However, it is not the whole story and simply taking oestrogen or testosterone replacement will not always fix it. Loss of libido is reflected through psychological feelings and relationship issues as well as hormonal ones and finding one cause for it is not always easy.

Psychological influences, such as how you approach ageing, thoughts about your body changing, and emotional closeness to your partner will all affect your desire for sex. HRT will sometimes help but is not always the answer.

Tips for improving desire:

◆ Address any physical issues – vaginal dryness, pain on lovemaking, bladder symptoms and your body image may need exploring.

◆ Encourage intimacy – for most women, it is emotional closeness that leads to the desire for sex. You may need to think about how to rebuild this, after years of taking it for granted, putting family first and the pressures of work and home.

◆ Communicate – talk to your partner about it. Assumptions and guesswork can lead to misunderstandings and taking the time to talk honestly about this important area will really help.

FSIAD

Female sexual interest/arousal disorder (FSIAD) is something different to acknowledging low feelings of desire and trying to find ways to improve the situation. It is when the lack of desire starts to cause physical or emotional distress to the extent that it impacts on your quality of life or causes problems in your relationship. Menopause, and all the associated physical, emotional and psychological effects of it, may contribute to difficulty in some women. There is no test or threshold to diagnose FSIAD; rather, it depends on how you individually are being affected. You may seek help from a doctor or sex therapist, who will address all the many issues that might be contributing to it, including, for some women, hormone replacement of oestrogen and sometimes testosterone.

Sexual infection

Have I really got to start all this again?

You might think that the 'safe sex' message is only for teenagers, but if you are starting a new relationship, it counts for you too. Sexual infections are on the rise among men and women over 40, as they start new relationships as a result of relationship breakdown,

Some causes of low libido

Physical causes	Psychological causes	Relationship causes
Hormonal changes – menopause	Other medical conditions, e.g. diabetes, disability or certain medications	Poor communication
Tiredness		Family changes
Vaginal discomfort or pain – oestrogen lack	Anxiety or stress	Changes in partner's health
Surgical – bladder or gynaecological surgery	Concerns about ageing and body image	Major life changes – divorce, redundancy, retirement
	Self-esteem issues and confidence	Changing social role
	Mental health concerns like depressions and anxiety	Satisfaction with relationship/partner

divorce or, sadly, death. A liberal attitude in society means that having new sexual partners is common, and both men and women may be exposed to the risk of sexual infection. If you are starting a new relationship, the advice is what you might offer your teenagers: 'Are you sure you are ready to have sex?' And: 'Be responsible', which now means protecting yourself against sexual infection with the use of condoms and, if in doubt, getting tested and remembering that a mutually monogamous relationship with a trusted partner will minimise risk.

Contraception: when can you stop?

One of the eventual freedoms of menopause is the release from the need to use contraception: but just when can you stop? You need to remember that while fertility declines with age pregnancies have been seen in women who thought they were menopausal and even after periods have apparently stopped. You may have irregular periods leading up to the menopause, sometimes for months at a time, and, with hormones fluctuating during this time, the chance of pregnancy is small but real.

If you are going through menopause at the usual time, at around 45 to 55 years, these are the recommendations:

◆ If you are under 50, you can stop contraception once you have not had a natural period for two years.

◆ If you are over 50, you can stop contraception once you have not had a natural period for one year.

If you are using hormonal contraception, which includes pills, injections, implants, some coils and contraceptive patches, or any type of HRT, your 'periods' are not entirely natural but influenced by the hormones, so you need to take extra care when thinking about stopping contraception. Your bleeding pattern may not give you a good indication as to what is happening with your hormones, so it will be difficult to know when to stop. With some of these methods, you may be able to have a blood test to help with the decision to stop contraception, but some, like the injection, may mask hormonal changes.

In this instance, you will usually be advised to continue using contraception until around 54 years, the age at which most women are post-menopausal. While you continue with contraception, you may want to change types. After the age of 50, you are likely to be advised to stop the combined contraceptive pill because of potential health risks and switch to a progestogen-only pill, coil (intrauterine), or condoms. See the Resource section for information about making contraception choices around the menopause.

If you go through menopausal changes very young, under the age of 40, and have 'premature ovarian insufficiency', you should discuss the need for contraception with your doctor. The need will depend on your age and the cause of the hormone deficiency.

Cancer screening for women

Cancer screening is when you have certain tests performed while you are healthy to detect any signs of cancer at a very early stage. Cancer screening saves lives and even prevents some cancers from developing because screening detects cell changes at such an early stage. Detecting cancers before they develop or at a very early stage improves the chances of successful treatment or even avoids the need for cancer treatment at all. This is an advantage of screening.

Screening for cancer is not perfect and can miss cancers, so you should not rely only on screening tests. You know your own body, and if you notice a change you should seek medical advice, even if you have had screening. Screening may mean that you have to come back for more tests, which may make you anxious, and sometimes screening may pick up signs of cancer that would never have grown at all or been very slow to develop. This is a disadvantage of screening.

In the UK there are three screening programmes for women. You need to be registered with a general practitioner to receive an invite for screening.

Cervical cancer screening

Cervical screening looks for changes in cells at the neck of the womb (cervix) using cytology, taking a sample of cells using a tiny brush. It involves an 'internal' examination, which, while not usually painful, may be uncomfortable, especially around the time of the menopause. Cervical screening is offered to women from the age of 25 until the age of 64, initially every three years and, from the age of 50, every five years. Hormonal changes after the menopause mean that sometimes you may get a result that is described as 'inadequate' and will need a repeat test. This may be a result of vaginal dryness, making the test difficult and cells hard to brush. You may be offered a short course of vaginal oestrogen in the lead up to the repeat test and then told to avoid using it for a few days before the test itself.

> **Recommendation**
>
> If you need vaginal oestrogen to make cervical screening more comfortable and effective, consider whether you might benefit from it long term, not just to get the screening done.

Breast cancer screening

Breast screening uses mammography, a type of X-Ray, to look at breast tissue and detect the early change in cells. In the UK you will be invited for breast screening at three-yearly intervals between the ages of 50 and 70 (at age 47 in some areas). If you are over 70 and wish to continue breast screening, you can do so by asking to stay in the recall system. Speak with your GP or local breast-screening unit. If you have a higher than average risk of breast cancer, for example, due to family history or inherited gene fault, you may be offered screening from a younger age.

You do not need more frequent breast screening just because you are on HRT.

Bowel screening

The NHS offers two types of screening for bowel cancer:

1. Faecal Occult Test (FOB). This tests for blood in your poo and you do the test in the privacy of your home, using a testing kit sent in the post. In England, Wales and Northern Ireland it is offered at two–yearly

intervals between the ages of 60 and 74. In Scotland, it is offered between the ages of 50 and 74 years.

2. Bowel scope. In England, this programme is being rolled out to men and women over the age of 55. It is a one-off test to look at polyps in the bowel, using a thin tube with a camera. Polyps don't usually cause symptoms but might turn into cancer if not removed. Most people do not find this test particularly uncomfortable although it is certainly not one you would want too often. Some find it embarrassing. Staff will help you relax and remember: it is a medical screen for your benefit that you only need once. It involves preparing the bowel in advance and you will be sent the information beforehand to do this. The actual bowel scope takes only five to ten minutes, and the whole appointment around half an hour.

Looking ahead

Menopause is a usually a natural stage in life. If you have no symptoms, it is about taking the time to improve health, to look ahead and make changes that will be steps towards preventing disease in the future and being well and healthy for the years beyond menopause. Perhaps it is a time of acceptance, of physical changes and life changes, but it is also a time of opportunities, a chance to be in control of your health and to look forward positively to the years ahead.

Frequently asked questions about health at menopause

1 *Is there such a thing as a 'menopause diet'?*

A healthy diet is always to be recommended and at menopause it is no different. There is no magic 'menopause diet' that does the job, just the usual advice both men and women should be following. In this chapter, you will find advice about healthy eating and in particular what, as a woman, you should be considering around menopause. You might, for example, want to consider whether your diet is worsening your symptoms: high caffeine intake, alcohol, and spicy food may all influence flushes.

2 *I have been smoking all my life. Is it even worth stopping now? Isn't it too late?*

It does not matter how old you are, or how long you have been smoking, you will always see a benefit to health by quitting. Your lungs and heart will function better, your risk of a heart attack will reduce and your risk of cancer will be lower. This chapter has advice about stopping smoking and the Resources chapter suggests more places to get help.

3 *I never go to the doctor. How often should I get my blood pressure checked?*

If you are not on any medicines and want to check your blood pressure periodically to be sure that it is healthy, once or twice a year is probably enough. You can check it at some pharmacies, gyms and health clubs as well as at your surgery.

4 *My mother had a heart attack in her fifties. Do I need any checks?*

You should discuss this with your doctor, who will make a cardiovascular risk assessment (as described in this chapter) and then let you know if you need any tests or specific advice in order to minimise your personal risk.

5 *I have heard that full-fat milk is better than skimmed for calcium. Is this true?*

In fact the calcium content of milk does not depend on its fat content: skimmed milk and low-fat dairy products have about as much calcium as full-fat equivalents. So if you switch to skimmed or semi-skimmed milk, you can be reassured that you are still getting the goodness of calcium. Half a pint of milk contains about 240g of calcium. Calcium is discussed in this chapter.

6 *I want to increase my exercise. How do I start?*

Start by looking at how you might build exercise more into your daily life. Could you take stairs more often, park further away, get off a bus stop sooner, or go for a walk at lunchtime? Then consider how you might increase exercise to build up to the level recommended for fitness and strength. Would you prefer to join a class or gym, or do an activity alone or with friends, like jogging or swimming? Look at what might be available locally and make your choice – than give it a go. Put it in your diary (mentally or actually!) and go for it. At first it might be hard, but build up gradually, both in terms of time and effort, and you will start to see the benefits over time. Keep in your mind the reasons you are doing it: is it to lose weight, to improve fitness or stamina? Is it to keep up with the children (or grandchildren) or simply for you, to keep healthy for longer? Remembering this helps to keep you motivated. See Resources section for links to tips and ideas about exercise on NHS websites.

7 *Should I get a bone scan?*

Not all women need a routine bone scan. If you think you may have a higher than usual risk for osteoporosis then you should discuss it with your doctor. You may like to use the risk calculator tool FRAX discussed in this chapter and outlined in the Resources section as well as reviewing other reasons why you think you might be at risk.

In the next chapter, I will consider how you can minimise the effects of menopausal symptoms without using HRT and then, in Chapter 4, we look at HRT.

chapter 3

Managing your symptoms without hormones

A different approach

Menopause is natural, I want to cope it with it naturally.

Why would I want to use hormones if I can manage without?

For most women, going through the menopause is a natural stage of life and one that they would prefer to do as naturally as possible. The 'medicalisation' of natural life events suggests that medical solutions are always the best whereas you may not want or need medical help. Some see the use of HRT as 'unnatural', although in Chapter 4 you will discover that HRT is more 'natural' than you may think. HRT is known to be effective but can be associated with certain side effects, so if you ask most women, they are likely to tell you that they would prefer to avoid hormones if they can. There have been so many myths and misunderstandings about hormone replacement therapy over the years that few women actively seek it without having tried other things first. The market for 'menopause relief' products has grown and if you go into a pharmacy or health-food shop, there will be shelf after shelf of products. If you have troublesome menopausal symptoms you might browse the shelves, wondering where to start.

Why no hormones?

Here are some of the reasons why you might not want to consider hormonal treatments:

- You believe that menopause is natural and want to keep it that way.
- Your symptoms may not warrant medical treatment, but you would like to try something that might help.
- You want to try something 'natural' first.
- You may have been advised to avoid HRT for medical reasons.
- You may be worried about using HRT, because of the side effects and risks you have read about.

Researching treatments

When you look at products and treatments that you can buy, how should you make a judgement as to whether or not something is worth using? Do you read the packet and hope it is true? Do you ask other women for their opinion or do you look at scientific evidence and make comparisons between products?

When your doctor chooses a medical treatment, they are guided by research studies over many years. Medical treatments including HRT are subject to strict licensing that requires there to be evidence of effectiveness and safety. These studies have been performed in large numbers of women over long periods of time and placebo controlled, which means comparing the hormonal treatment with a placebo (dummy) medicine to see if the benefits can be fully attributed to the treatment and not to chance. Usually, one particular group of symptoms is assessed, most commonly flushes and sweats as they can be fairly easily measured in an objective way. Doses of HRT used in the studies have to reflect everyday use and the evidence can often easily be compared from one HRT to another. This approach works for medicines that have to be strictly tested to ensure safety and to show that they work. Claims made by medicines must be accurate and supported by medical research. In the UK, the MHRA (Medicines and Healthcare Products Regulatory Agency) carefully supervises this and monitors any adverse or unwanted effects from licensed medications.

The issue becomes more complex with regard to complementary and alternative approaches. The manufacturers do not make medical claims for their products, but make more general statements instead, like 'may help with menopause', 'for women going through menopause', or 'useful at the time of menopause'. Such products do not require objective studies to prove any benefits but this does not necessarily mean that they are ineffective or unsafe. If studies have been done, they might be studies of short duration, not placebo controlled, and may not use the same dose as the one in the product on the shelf. Some products will have a broader base of scientific research than others, so we know more about these and can be more confident about their benefits. Many of the products are a combination of components making it even harder to assess if any of the single constituents has a real benefit.

The science

I'd like to know if they really do work, before spending my money.

If you look at independent scientific data relating to non-medical products you often see that the comment 'insufficient evidence' is made. This means that the body of scientists investigating the claim could not find enough studies of a sufficiently high scientific standard to include in the review. Smaller studies may have had positive results but these cannot be assumed to apply to all women. So finding the evidence to check these treatments out may be difficult. Herbal products in the UK, but not food supplements, do have to submit evidence to regulatory authorities that the product contains precisely what it claims to, that it has been used historically for this condition, and that there is safety data supporting its use. They do not, however, have to show scientific evidence that they are effective in what they claim to be used for. So this is different from conventional medicines, including HRT. Vitamins, multivitamins and other food supplements are not subject to this same check, and standardisation and quality of ingredients vary across manufacturers. Buying from reputable suppliers, rather than unknown ones, will help with quality assurance. In particular, you should be cautious about buying from overseas internet sites, where you may not be able to verify either the product content or its source.

What women say

It worked for my friend, so I thought I would give it a try.

Many of the products will carry endorsements from women who claim to have benefited from it. These are valid endorsements but reflect only their personal experience. You may try the product and find it of no benefit. For most women, menopausal symptoms will eventually improve of their own accord and this might coincide with taking a particular product, which means that you attribute it to that. In HRT studies it has been demonstrated that even women in the placebo arm, that is taking a dummy medicine, got some degree of improvement in symptoms but not to the same extent or for as long as the active HRT. Some would argue that the placebo effect of starting a treatment that you hope will work, and have probably paid for, often does give some initial relief. The real test is: does it last? Others would say: does it matter if it is only a placebo effect? If you feel better and it does no harm, that is a result. The answer lies with you. Do you want to take something that has substantial evidence to say it works and is backed by medical research or have you reached the point where anything is worth a try as long as it is not harmful? Are you open to it working for a bit and then symptoms returning, perhaps suggesting a placebo effect? That is a decision for you to make.

Why it is difficult for doctors to recommend herbal products

I asked my doctor about alternatives, but he said nothing's as good as HRT. That might be true, but I don't want HRT.

Apparently 'natural' is not necessarily safer.

Healthcare professionals have to work from an evidence and safety basis. They have a responsibility to ensure that anything they recommend has a good base of science behind it in order to ensure both safety and efficacy. This is to protect you, the patient, and to make sure that in the NHS at least, only treatments which are tried, tested and safe are used. This means that they tend to stick to advising about conventional medicines where such evidence is freely available and may sometimes be accused of only taking a 'medical' approach. There are some non-hormonal treatments that can be prescribed (see below) but once you start using herbal treatments and supplements then you are treating yourself rather than being treated. Some call this the 'natural' approach, although you do need to be careful. 'Natural' products may have side effects, and unwanted effects too, and, more importantly, may sometimes interact with other medical treatments you are using.

In this chapter, I will look at common groups of menopausal symptoms and suggest ways of alleviating them without using HRT. This will include the following:

◆ Lifestyle changes to manage symptoms

◆ Herbal or dietary supplements

◆ Cognitive behavioural therapy

◆ Therapy approaches, e.g. acupuncture

◆ Non-hormonal medicines your doctor might prescribe.

Flushes and sweats

Hot flushes and night sweats, the most common menopausal symptoms, often come and go and will eventually stop of their own accord. They will often last for up to about five years, but a few women will see them go on for much longer than this, occasionally seeming as if they will never go away, and they can still happen in your sixties and beyond. Sometimes there are factors that will trigger them or worsen their intensity, so identifying these may help you to minimise their effects:

◆ Caffeine and spicy foods

◆ Alcohol

◆ Smoking

◆ Intense exercise

◆ Feeling pressured for time or anxious

◆ Moving from different temperatures, e.g. room to room, having a hot bath, or even using a hairdryer.

Try these tips to help you get through flushes:

◆ Wear layers of clothes, so that you can easily slip one

off when you start to feel hot. Avoid high neck or close fitting clothes if you feel warm around the neck.

◆ Smoking may worsen them, so this is another good reason to cut back.

◆ Keep wipes or body spray handy to cool down and freshen up. Try cooling sprays, which mainly aim to cool you in the midst of a flush.

◆ If stress is a trigger, consider yoga or relaxation-type exercises.

◆ Position fans at work or home to keep cool air circulating.

◆ Remember to drink plenty of water.

◆ Keep your bedroom cool, turn down the heat and perhaps sleep on a towel, so that you can easily change it if you wish.

◆ Consider using a cooling pack under your pillow then turning the pillow regularly.

◆ Allow yourself more time: flushes often worsen when you feel under pressure.

Some everyday foods and drinks are known to trigger flushes in some women at the time of menopause so consider these recommendations:

◆ Reduce caffeine intake over the day.

◆ Alcohol – consider cutting out that late-night glass of wine and reduce alcohol generally.

◆ Spicy foods sometimes make flushes worse.

You may find that making small adjustments like these does make a difference to how much the flushes bother you, so consider keeping a diary and noting what for you are the worse triggers.

Gadgets and aids for flushes

You will see various items advertised that are intended to make life easier if you have flushes and sweats. While these do not treat the symptoms, you may find them helpful as they aim primarily to make you feel cooler at the moment of a flush or sweat. Such items include purpose-made cooling pads, cooling mists, bed linen with cooling properties, and even clothing aimed at women who need to constantly put on and take off layers because of flushes. Don't underestimate the benefits, too, of a handbag mini-fan and a desk fan – simple things that help in the moment of that flush to make you feel more comfortable.

Supplements for flushes

There are many products sold to women that supposedly reduce flushes and you may want to see if they work for you. With regard to those that have some medical evidence to support their use, the following may be worth considering. In all supplements, individual products vary widely in what they contain and in the actual doses, so do your research and look for brands that are clear on content and standardisation.

In the UK, the health organisation NICE (National Institute for Health and Care Excellence) has reviewed the scientific data for supplements suggested for menopause and concluded that there is mixed evidence and that black cohosh and isoflavones may help flushes and sweats.

Black cohosh. This potent herb, also called *Actaea racemosa*, has been used for many years to help menopausal symptoms. It has been widely researched and if used at the low doses available in the UK (40 mg) is considered to be low risk and with few side effects. Black cohosh may work in the body in a similar way to oestrogen, so you are advised not to use it if you cannot use HRT, if, for example, you have had breast or womb cancer. Black cohosh may interact with some medicines so if you use regular medications you should check with your doctor before using it. You should not use black cohosh if you have had liver damage and, as it is not entirely known how it works, you should avoid it if you have had breast cancer.

Isoflavones. These are various types of phytoestrogens, plant-derived substances that in some ways mimic oestrogen in chemical structure and effect. Soybeans and soya products are the richest source of isoflavones in diet and are found in food such as soya milk, chickpeas and tofu. There is some evidence that, taken as dietary supplements or through diet, they can help hot flushes. Natural isoflavones can also be found in red clover and this is available as a dietary supplement at doses of 40 mg and 80 mg. If you have had breast cancer, speak to your doctor before using red clover or any other isoflavone supplement.

It is likely that supplements will take a while to work and you may need to use them for three months before you notice any particular benefit. Bear this in mind when you look at costs.

Alternative ideas for flushes

Other women will sometimes champion products which are not supported by clinical evidence in terms of their effectiveness in relieving hot flushes. That does not mean that individual women do not sincerely believe that they work, simply that, when subjected to clinical research, no objective benefits could be seen. Nonetheless, you might decide to try them anyway. Such alternatives include:

◆ Magnets
◆ Sage
◆ Evening primrose oil
◆ Dong quai
◆ Gingko.

> ### Recommendation
>
> Remember that any active herb or supplement that is potent enough to be effective might be strong enough to do harm. If you take regular medication, be aware that there may be an interaction, and if in doubt seek medical advice before starting.

Conventional medicines without hormones for flushes

I tried all the alternatives, but finally turned back to my doctor even though I knew I could not use HRT.

If you are struggling to cope with flushes and sweats and cannot use HRT, your doctor may suggest other medicines which are not hormones. Your doctor may want you to see a specialist before using some of these because some are being used 'off licence'. That means that they are licensed as a medicine for a different condition and have been shown to have the added benefit of helping flushes in some women. Doctors commonly use medicines in this way and should explain to you when this is the case, and if they are not familiar themselves with using a medicine off licence they should refer you on to someone who is. Specialists working in a particular therapeutic area, such as a menopause specialist or cancer specialist, may see many women using medicines in this way, whereas a GP will see very few.

Clonidine

Clonidine is a long-standing licensed non-hormonal treatment for flushes. Women sometimes say that it works initially and then stops working; others find it beneficial. The usual advice is to stop clonidine if you have not noticed any benefit after using it for around four weeks. Clonidine lowers blood pressure, so if you have been using it for more than about four weeks it is usually advised that you taper it off, reducing the dose over a couple of weeks before stopping.

SSRIS and SNRIS

At first, I did not want to consider antidepressants, but once I understood why it was being offered, I gave them a try.

Selective serotonin reuptake inhibitors and serotonin-norepinephrine reuptake inhibitors are both types of medicine used as antidepressants or for anxiety. When used at low doses, they have been suggested for relief of hot flushes, although the exact way they work is unclear. They have been widely researched and in some women show a benefit that is greater than using nothing (placebo) and not as great as using standard dose HRT. They start to work quite quickly, so a short course is usually enough to find out if it will work for you: often a two- to four-week trial is offered at first. Side effects may occur in the first few days and may include dry mouth, sleep disturbance and nausea, all of which usually settles with time. If you are offered antidepressants for flushes, your doctor does not necessarily think that you are depressed. These drugs are now being prescribed for flushes, but as they are not licensed for this particular symptom there will be nothing relevant in the information leaflet to help you.

> **Recommendation**
>
> If you are using tamoxifen, you should avoid SSRIs, e.g. paroxetine and fluoxetine, because of potential interaction with tamoxifen. You can, however, use citalopram and SNRIs, e.g. venlafaxine.

Gabapentin

My specialist breast doctor suggested this as my flushes were just so bad.

Gabapentin is an analogue of gamma-aminobutyric acid and is generally used to treat pain or seizures. Sometimes it helps with flushes. Your doctor will start at a low dose and gradually work up to a higher dose in order to avoid side effects such as nausea and dizziness. Gabapentin is more likely to be suggested in a specialist clinic, where the doctors use it more regularly for this purpose, and is often reserved for women who have medical reasons for avoiding HRT.

Cognitive behavioural therapy (CBT)

I feel out of control; this will go on forever.

Cognitive behaviour therapy is a brief, non-medical approach that can be helpful for a range of health problems. It has been suggested for anxiety and stress, depressed mood, hot flushes and night sweats, sleep problems and fatigue. CBT can help you develop practical ways of managing problems and provides new coping skills and useful strategies. For this reason, it can be a helpful approach to consider because the skills can be applied to different problems, and can therefore improve well-being in general.

Professor Myra Hunter, a clinical and academic psychologist with King's College, London, has developed a CBT approach for menopausal symptoms that has been found to be effective in several clinical trials. She has produced a fact sheet (available on www.womens-health-concern.org) and a self-help manual for women – see the Resources section. The information below on CBT, including the diagrams, has been summarised from Professor Hunter's work, with her permission.

Self-help with CBT

Anxiety and stress are common reactions to everyday life. The menopause is not necessarily a stressful time but it occurs during midlife when you may be dealing with other life challenges, such as parents' ill-health or bereavement, adolescent children, children leaving home (or not leaving home), or work demands. Having hot flushes and night sweats can also be stressful, and being anxious and stressed can make hot flushes more difficult to deal with.

Stress usually happens when we are in a situation that seems too demanding or overwhelming and we think that we don't have the personal resources to deal with it – we start to think that we can't cope, which then adds to the stress. When we feel stressed or under threat, the body releases adrenaline to quickly send blood and oxygen to the muscles so that they are prepared for action. Our breathing becomes faster in order to take in more oxygen, and muscles tense to help the body fight or run. This response is not very adaptive in modern life, when most of our stresses are not life-threatening, such as being late or facing pressure at work. If you have many demands in your daily life, this stress response can be constantly activated. While this is not dangerous, over time it can build up and affect health and well-being. Similarly, anxiety is a normal reaction to threatening situations, but it becomes problematic when benign and non-dangerous situations and events are regularly perceived as threats, which is more likely to happen if you feel stressed. So reducing anxiety and stress is a helpful strategy that will improve well-being and will minimise the impact of stress on menopausal symptoms in your daily life.

CBT for anxiety and stress focuses on the links between physical symptoms, thoughts, feelings and behaviour. The way we think about symptoms in certain situations tends to affect how we feel and what we do, and these reactions can in turn increase the intensity of bodily reactions.

Cognitive and behavioural strategies can be used to develop a calmer or accepting view of a situation and therefore to respond (behave) in a helpful way. If you feel anxious or stressed, write down your thoughts, feelings and behavioural reactions following the example of the diagram on page 96. Once you have identified a typical

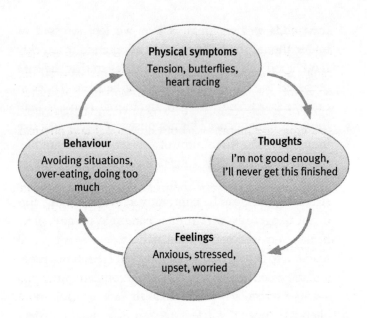

anxious thought, consider whether it is overly negative, overestimating the threat, or underestimating your ability to cope. Remember – anxious/stressful thoughts are not facts but are just one view of a situation. Ask yourself: is there really a threat? What would a calm person think in this situation? What would you say to a close friend if they were in this situation? Have I managed similar situations before? Check your behavioural responses to anxiety and stress and if you are over-working, eating/drinking too much, or avoiding certain people or activities, then consider more helpful alternatives.

Low mood and menopause

CBT for low mood is helpful for people across the age range and when physical and emotional symptoms occur together. As for anxiety, low mood and hot flushes often occur together and the cognitive and behavioural strategies are helpful for both emotional and physical symptoms.

When people are depressed, they tend to think more negatively about themselves and the world in general and have negative expectations about the future. Depressive thinking and behaviour can lead to a cycle of self-criticism and hopelessness, as shown in the diagram below, and many people often withdraw and avoid situations, feeling worse as a result. This can

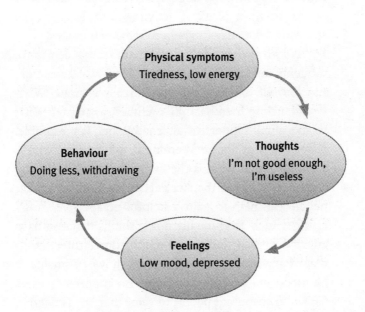

happen to people who would normally think quite differently when they are not depressed. CBT can help people to identify overly negative thoughts so that they can gain a perspective on their concerns and gradually learn how to manage these thoughts.

Cognitive and behavioural strategies can help people to make changes so that they begin to increase activity and be less self-critical. The first step is to look at life from a broad perspective – the things that you value (about yourself and life in general), what you used to enjoy doing, and/or how you would like things to be in five years' time. Then you could gradually re-engage in activities that you previously valued and enjoyed but which you might have dropped or withdrawn from since feeling low. Making these changes in behaviour by engaging in pleasant activities and developing a structure to the day can help to initially lift mood.

As with anxiety and stress, remember that depressive thoughts are not facts but are just one view of a situation. Ask yourself: is this view of myself really accurate? What would a close friend/family member say to me? What would a self-supportive alternative be? For example, instead of 'I'm not good enough', ask yourself who is saying this and what is the evidence – we are usually harder on ourselves than we need to be. Talking to other people can help to gain a helpful perspective. Small changes such as gradually doing things that you have enjoyed, or new things, and writing down three things that went well at the end of each day (however small) can lift mood and improve well-being. An important part of CBT is to encourage people to value their own qualities, strengths and competencies. If problems are persistent, for example financial, health, housing and so on, then 'problem-solve', considering all options with someone else, and seek practical help and advice.

CBT for hot flushes focuses on the links between physical symptoms, thoughts, feelings and behaviour. The way we think about symptoms in certain situations tends to affect the emotions we feel and what we do, and these reactions can in turn increase the intensity of the hot flushes.

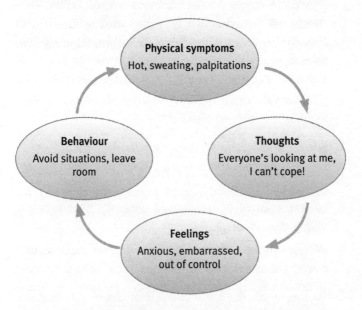

For example, as shown in the diagram above, when this woman feels the onset of a hot flush, she thinks that everyone is looking at her and that she can't cope; this leads to feelings of embarrassment, loss of control and anxiety. These feelings might then lead to increased tension, palpitations and sweating, which intensify the hot flush experience. CBT can help you to find ways to reduce these negative reactions to hot flushes. Learning calmer more neutral responses will help you to feel more in control and more able to cope.

Cognitive and behavioural strategies

Paced breathing is an important part of the CBT approach for hot flushes. As with any skill it requires regular practice. At the onset of a flush, relax your shoulders, breathe slowly from your stomach and concentrate on your breathing. Paced breathing involves focusing on your breath, accepting that the hot flush will pass, and just letting the hot flush flow over you.

Women's main types of worries about hot flushes and night sweats tend to be:

1. Social embarrassment (especially around men, younger people, and at work): 'Everyone's looking at me', 'I look terrible'.

2. Lack of control: 'This is out of control', 'I can't cope with these', 'Not again!'

3. Worries about disrupted sleep : 'I'll never get back to sleep', 'I'll feel terrible tomorrow'.

Women with the highest levels of distress in reaction to hot flushes tend to 'catastrophise' about the hot flush, that is, think the worst. They are more self-critical within the situation, especially about their appearance. Notice what goes through your mind when you have a hot flush, so that you can identify your typical thoughts and any overly negative thinking, and write them down.

Next, work on developing a calmer, self-supporting response to hot flushes, for example, 'This will pass soon', 'I will notice my flushes more than other people, they may not notice' , 'Let's see how well I can deal with this one, one flush at a time'.

It might help to ask yourself: Is my thinking really accurate? What would a close friend/family member say to me? What would I say to them if they were having a hot flush in this situation? What would a self-supportive alternative be?

How to access CBT

The delivery of CBT will vary from an online resource to telephone support to face-to-face counselling and may be available in some form on the NHS, but sometimes with a long waiting time. Details of Professor Hunter's self-help guide are in the Resources chapter.

Other kinds of therapy

Taking time out for me, with a registered practitioner offering an individual therapy, has been so helpful, I feel ready to face the world again.

Some women turn to other therapies for help with flushes, for example, acupuncture, reflexology, mindfulness and massage. Therapists who offer treatments like these are not usually looking to treat specific symptoms but to treat you individually and with tailored treatment to look after your 'whole being'. This makes it difficult to conduct studies to examine the effectiveness of treatments as the bottom line may not be 'do you have fewer flushes' but 'is life any easier?'. Using therapies such as these is sometimes described as an 'integrated approach', where you may combine a therapy such as acupuncture with dietary and lifestyle changes. Taking this approach may improve a sense of well-being at a time when symptoms are particularly bothersome. This is difficult to measure, so clinical trials are difficult to do, but some women will describe benefit from this approach. Some points to consider when choosing to use therapies include:

- Look up the professional body which regulates that particular therapy, if there is one, and ask your practitioner if they are registered, e.g. British Acupuncture Society, Association of Reflexologists. Others are mentioned in the Resources chapter.

- Ask questions before committing to treatment: how many sessions will be suggested, how much will they cost, what is the expected benefit? How long will you continue treatment?

- Check the therapist's qualifications and ask if they have insurance.

- Where will they see you? Remember that you will be in a private room with an unknown individual. Exercise caution.

Mood swings and emotional changes

It is the up- and down-ness that troubles me; one day fine, the next tearful or angry.

You may notice your variation in moods more acutely as you go through menopause. Whereas you used to feel on an even keel you now feel a little unpredictable in your responses, and others might be saying that you have changed a bit, perhaps become a bit more irritable or tetchy. This can lead to misunderstandings at home or work, sometimes leading to anxiety and stress in situations where you would usually feel in control. Your menopausal symptoms may contribute to changes in mood, so addressing those is one step towards helping this issue.

Tips for improving menopausal mood:

◆ Stay active – regular exercise lifts mood and improves energy levels. Blood flow to the brain and body improves, which may help 'brain fog'.

◆ Don't isolate yourself – you may feel like shutting out friends and family, but this can lower mood further. Try to tell your partner or friends how you feel. Consider joining a forum where shared voices sometimes help (e.g., menopausematters.co.uk – see the Resources chapter).

◆ Consider counselling or cognitive therapy approaches.

◆ Positive framing – it is easy to look at the negatives, but try looking at the good things in your life. Focus on these when you feel low and it may help your mood.

◆ Challenge negative attitudes to menopause. Society tells us we have to stay young-looking but look around you; the average menopausal woman can be healthy, active and have many roles in life.

◆ Relax – consider mindfulness, relaxation classes or yoga, and take back time for yourself in a busy week.

◆ Plan your pleasures – don't feel guilty about making time for yourself, whether it is coffee with friends or, if finances allow, booking a holiday.

Herbals

The supplement St John's wort has traditionally been used to treat low mood. It is reported to work like standard antidepressants but with fewer side effects and in a milder way. You should not take St John's wort if you already use an antidepressant and should be cautious if using sleeping tablets. St John's wort reduces the effectiveness of some contraceptive pills, so speak to your doctor if you are on the pill form of contraceptive. If you have had breast cancer and are using tamoxifen, it is advisable not to use St John's wort as it may render the tamoxifen less effective.

As with all herbals, you need to consider the product you buy since doses and types will vary. In the UK, St John's wort products will carry the registration mark of a traditional herbal therapy, which ensures a product that meets standardisation and safety requirements.

Tiredness, lack of energy and poor sleep

I get home from work and all I want to do is flop on the sofa – I have absolutely no energy.

You may feel more tired than normal, and some describe an exhaustion that seems unrelenting. It is difficult to know if these are directly related to hormonal changes or other symptoms contributing to this: night sweats might be keeping you up at night, for example. Stress may be a contributing factor along with anxiety or depression.

Tips for improving tiredness:

- Think about your sleep habits – review your night-time routine.
- Avoid 'screen time' close to bed time – this means TV, phone, laptops and iPads.
- Increase exercise – this seems counterintuitive but it will raise your energy levels and promote endorphin production. Try a lunchtime walk to improve daytime energy.
- Try relaxation techniques to reduce stress.
- Reduce caffeine and alcohol intake, especially at night – both may disrupt sleep as well as worsen flushes.
- Stay hydrated during the day.
- Consider over-the-counter sleep aids, such as valerian or lavender oil.
- Address issues like anxiety and depression, seeking help if necessary.

> **Recommendation**
>
> If you suffer profound exhaustion and can see no obvious cause, seek medical advice to rule out medical conditions such as thyroid condition or anaemia.

Poor concentration and forgetfulness

The words go in, I am listening ... but recalling it is a problem. This is new. I used to recall everything really well.

I can be in the middle of a sentence and just forget what I am saying; I just lose my train of thought.

Poor memory and concentration can affect your work as well as your home life. You may feel overloaded when facing too many tasks and embarrassed when you forget things. This may be caused by the changes in oestrogen levels and helped by HRT, but lack of sleep may contribute and trying to hold down multiple responsibilities may make it worse. Treatment of underlying causes, like stress, anxiety or poor sleep, will help, along with acknowledging the effects and addressing them with simple strategies:

- Lists, reminders and diaries – more now than ever!
- Try not to allow time pressures to build – give yourself more time to complete reports and reading.
- Consider supplements such as isoflavones, Bach flower remedies, gingko biloba or vitamin B complex, all anecdotally reported to improve memory.

Vaginal dryness and painful sex

Lovemaking became so painful, I would avoid it, going to bed first, pretending to be asleep.

My partner was patient, but in the end, I knew I had to do something to improve it.

Vaginal dryness can be more than just a nuisance. As oestrogen levels fall during and after menopause, dryness, soreness, itching and painful sex are very common symptoms yet are seldom discussed. Not just related to sex, vaginal dryness can lead to discomfort at any time as well as itching and pain. Vaginal oestrogen will treat the underlying cause, and there are non-hormonal solutions to treat the symptoms for those women who want to avoid hormones. The advantage of non-hormonals is that you do not have to see a doctor, simply buy it online or at the pharmacy. Some women use low-dose vaginal oestrogen and a non-hormonal therapy to get the maximum benefit.

Moisturisers and lubricants

This made such a difference, in fact, the lubrication was better than before!

Finding it in the chemist was not easy, it's not something you want to go and ask about is it?

There is some overlap with these products as women often use the same for both purposes but there are differences. You may need to experiment with several products to find the one that is best for you.

Moisturisers are meant to be regularly used, usually two to three times a week, and help to 'cushion' the wall of the vagina by moisturising the tissue, making it softer and so less sore. They also have a positive effect on vaginal pH, which promotes natural 'good' bacteria, preventing thrush and similar infections. A vaginal moisturiser aims to replenish moisture and alleviate ongoing discomfort caused by the dryness. They are designed to be longer-lasting than lubricants so that with regular use, the symptoms of vaginal dryness improve. Vaginal moisturisers will improve general vaginal dryness symptoms often not associated with sex itself, so you may still need a lubricant before sex.

Lubricants aim to make lovemaking more comfortable by improving wetness and smoothness in the vagina, thus reducing friction that can lead to pain. They are designed to be short-lasting and to be used every time you make love. They can be inserted with applicators or using fingers inside the entrance of the vagina (or on the man's penis), and the amount you use can be adjusted as you get used to what you find helpful. Some women use lubricants regularly as a type of moisturiser to soothe dryness because they are pleasant and convenient to use, and also help to keep the vaginal pH comfortable.

Examples of vaginal moisturisers:

◆ Replens
◆ Yes VM
◆ Regelle.

Examples of lubricants:

◆ Sylk
◆ Yes
◆ Pjurmed.

Peer support and forums

It is so good to see that I am not alone, others have similar experiences.

I thought I was going crazy; to see other women saying exactly the same is so reassuring.

When you go through menopause, you sometimes feel isolated and unsure of yourself. Is this menopause? Are my symptoms typical or am I odd? Is this really menopause anyway?

Online you will find women contributing to forums and discussing their menopause. It is always important to remember that everyone is different and that you will read all kinds of stories and experiences. Go to reliable websites (some are mentioned in the Resources section of this book) and be open-minded, noting that absolutely anyone can write anything they want on these sites. Not all sites are moderated so double-check any medical advice that is offered. You may find it reassuring to read of other women's experiences and see that your symptoms are remarkably common. You may be willing to share your experience and help others in that way.

In some areas, you will find support groups and

local networks that can be very helpful. Often led by women, they can help you understand the changes that are occurring and point you in the direction of medical help if needed. Be aware that these are often voluntary groups led by enthusiastic volunteers rather than medical professionals and although some will have extended their understanding and knowledge of the topic, others will be working more to offer peer support than education or advice. Some have made great efforts to be fully educated on all aspects of menopause, others will simply work within the knowledge of their own menopause experience on a peer-support basis. All have a place: just be sure that you know which type of group it is. Look at the credentials of the leader.

Menopause mentors/coaches

Having someone to talk with, to share my goals and discuss a way of achieving them, was so helpful to me.

It helped me to sort out in my mind what is important and what I can let go of.

Some life coaches have specifically broadened their remit to include menopause life coaching, or 'menopause mentoring'. Life coaching is different to counselling or advising. Coaching is about listening and providing tools to cope with difficult situations, enabling you to make positive changes in your life. Life coaches encourage personal development through a given situation rather than trying to find a solution to it. They will not offer treatment or advice about medical conditions but will help you navigate your life through your experience of a particular condition; in this case, menopause. Life coaching is unregulated in the UK although many coaches will have evidence of membership of a recognised professional body, along with relevant qualifications and insurance cover. Life coaching can be done on a face-to-face basis, by telephone or online, and usually involves committing to a course of at least six sessions in advance. Life coaching or mentorship for menopause is an approach to coping with your symptoms and may be useful. It is important to remember that, however knowledgeable she may be, the life coach or mentor should not be offering individual medical advice.

This takes us back to the fact that menopause is a normal, natural event and not one that will always need medical intervention. Non-medical approaches should not replace HRT for those women who need it, either because they are young or because they have symptoms that restrict work and home life. Rather, as with any life event, there are options available to make it easier and strategies to cope. Achieving a healthy menopause means finding the right way for you, whether that is HRT or a non-medical approach.

Frequently asked questions about managing menopause without HRT

1 *Which is the best supplement to take at the time of the menopause?*

There is no single supplement that will quickly resolve symptoms or improve health around menopause. Consider if you want a supplement to try to resolve a specific symptom, such as flushes or sweats, in which case you might want to try one that has some evidence to support its use (see earlier in this chapter), or if you are looking for dietary support, because you might lack a particular nutrient, e.g. calcium or vitamin D. Do your research and check the doses on the packet, and make sure that you buy from a reputable source to ensure high quality and standardisation. If you are using conventional medicine, check that there will be no unwanted interactions.

2 *My doctor offered me antidepressants but I am not depressed. Is he fobbing me off?*

HRT is an effective treatment for many menopausal symptoms, but occasionally there are medical reasons why you should not use it (see Chapter 4). If you cannot use HRT, you may be offered an antidepressant at a low dose, as for some women, it can have a beneficial effect on flushes and sweats. It is not because your doctor believes you are depressed or wants to 'fob you off', but because of the 'added benefits' the drug may offer. You might be surprised to be offered antidepressants if you are not depressed but it is a reasonable choice in this instance.

3 *I have had breast cancer and cannot use HRT. My flushes on tamoxifen are awful, so can I try the supplements discussed in this chapter?*

You need to be cautious because some of them may work a little like a hormone and others may interact with your tamoxifen. Either way, if you are on tamoxifen, you should check with a health professional before using supplements for flushes. There may be non-hormonal medicines you could discuss with your doctor which may be a better option (see earlier in this chapter).

4 *Can I use over-the-counter vaginal preparations if I have had breast cancer?*

Vaginal moisturisers and lubricants that are available without prescription do not contain any hormones, so you may use these after breast cancer. See earlier in this chapter for a discussion about the difference between a moisturiser and a lubricant: both may be useful.

5 *I am sore inside the vagina but am not very comfortable with using my fingers to insert these (vaginal) products. What do you suggest?*

Some of the lubricants and moisturisers are packaged in tiny tubes so that you can insert it more easily, squeezing the product through a small applicator rather than using your fingers. If your partner is male, he can apply the lubricant to him, just before penetration.

6 *Can I use homeopathy to treat my symptoms?*

There are few studies looking at homeopathy for menopause symptoms and it is hard to know whether any benefits are truly treatment-related or can be attributed to the ongoing support such treatment practitioners offer. You should choose a qualified practitioner or homeopathic doctor if you consider it, and bear in mind the cost, like any private treatment.

7 *I have gone through natural menopause and feel fine; I just want to do my best to stay that way. Should I take HRT even though I don't have any symptoms?*

HRT is primarily given for treatment of menopausal symptoms or to protect health for those who are younger than average (under 45). Even though HRT has potential benefits to health, it is unlikely that you would be offered it if you don't have any symptoms and have gone though menopause at the usual age. As research and understanding of HRT improves, that might change in the future, perhaps for women with higher than average risk of heart disease or osteoporosis.

The next chapter looks at HRT in depth and how it is used. Even if you are fairly sure that HRT is not for you, I encourage you to read this chapter; you might be surprised by some of the information and will learn more about HRT benefits as well as the drawbacks of hormone treatment.

chapter 4

Hormone replacement therapy (HRT)

I was scared of trying HRT; there has been so much negative publicity.

I feel a failure because I needed HRT, it means I couldn't cope.

HRT has changed my life; at last, I feel normal.

You will have heard all sorts of things about HRT. Some of this will be true; some will be myth; and some will be partly right or will consist of a mixed-up message. Over the last fifteen years or so HRT has been subjected to numerous studies and scientific investigations and, each time, the media chooses how to portray the results. Sensational news is usually negative; the good news stories about HRT seldom make the headlines. You would hope that your doctor or healthcare professional would understand the data and would help you but in fact they too have been confused by it all. It can be hard to interpret the studies and developments happen so frequently that, unless you have a special interest in this area of health, you may not be up to date with or understand all of the new data, even as a health professional. Now that guidance has been issued to healthcare professionals from the National Institute for Health and Care Excellence (NICE) in the UK, it should be simpler for doctors and others to gather the information they need to tell you about HRT. You can find details of the NICE Guidance in the Resources chapter.

Why might you want HRT?

I reluctantly chose HRT, but my symptoms were getting me down so much.

I chose HRT because I wanted to be in control more of my life and my emotions.

I didn't really want HRT, but I had tried everything else.

Very few women actually want HRT; it is more a case of deciding that your symptoms are affecting life to such a degree that you are willing to try it. Maybe you are just not sleeping, troubled by flushes and sweats each and every night, maybe you are struggling to work effectively, your concentration is poor, you are tired, irritable and moody. Perhaps it feels like this menopause is just going on too long and you want to address it. Maybe those around you have noticed your symptoms and are concerned for you, suggesting you seek medical help. These are all valid reasons to consider the benefits for you of HRT.

I went through menopause at 41; HRT was strongly recommended.

It may be that you are going through menopause before

the age of 45, a bit younger than usual, or even much younger than that, and are advised to use HRT for the long-term health benefits as well as for symptom relief. You want to know more about it and what it involves.

What is HRT?

I assumed it was like the pill …

I wasn't really sure what was involved in taking HRT.

When we talk about HRT, we are referring to the use of hormones, such as oestrogen, progestogen (or progesterone) and sometimes testosterone, to treat symptoms of the menopause when it occurs naturally, or to counteract the effects of loss of the same hormones at a young age. It is quite different from 'the pill', the oral contraceptive: the type of hormone is different, the potency or strength is very different, and the effects are also different. That means that you cannot compare the pill to HRT, in terms of side effects or who can use it. You may have been advised not to use the contraceptive pill, but that does not necessarily mean that you cannot use HRT. Oestrogens used in HRT are closer to those produced naturally by you during your natural cycle and do not cause your levels of hormones to rise significantly above that which would be considered normal. The higher doses of synthetic oestrogen in the contraceptive pill are needed to suppress natural ovarian function and to be effective as contraception. HRT is not contraception and does not contain synthetic oestrogen.

Benefits of HRT

Symptoms

Within two or three weeks, I saw a reduction in my sweats – I slept at last.

It took a while, but looking back, I can see I am functioning better and am less tired.

I wish I had started it earlier, it has made such a difference to how I feel.

The main reason that you are likely to want HRT is to treat troublesome symptoms of the menopause. Maybe you have tried other alternatives, but the symptoms persist, and perhaps they are so bothersome that you feel the time has come to get medical help. HRT is the most effective treatment available for symptoms that arise due to menopause. Flushes and sweats will improve; you may sleep better, so symptoms like mood fluctuations, poor concentration and irritability may also improve. Low mood and muscle pains may improve with HRT too. Vaginal dryness improves so that sex becomes more enjoyable. If it is enjoyable, your desire for sex increases and so on. Skin and hair may improve in appearance, although do not expect to turn the clock back. When menopause occurs at the usual time of around age 50, it coincides with a lot of physical changes occurring because of ageing and HRT will not always address these. Taking HRT is not about staying youthful, but about staying healthy and functioning fully at work and home.

Symptoms like flushes and sweats should improve quite quickly, starting within a couple of weeks, although they may be slow to go completely. Symptoms like low mood, tiredness and poor concentration may take longer and will not suddenly improve. You will look back over the past couple of months and notice that things have got better rather than noticing a sudden improvement. Sometimes the dose might need adjusting to get maximum benefit so, after around three months, you can assess how you feel and make that decision with your prescriber.

Bones

My bone scan showed I was at risk of fracture later in life, so it is good to know that while treating my symptoms it is also good for that.

I am only 41 years old, so one of the reasons I take HRT is so that my bones are protected from osteoporosis.

Bone loss is a natural consequence of ageing and of menopause (see Chapter 1). Whether or not you are at risk of osteoporosis later in life will depend on many factors, but an important one is the age at which you go through menopause. Taking HRT at the time of the menopause, whenever that is, will help to stop the accelerated bone loss due to hormone changes. For young women, under 40, it is considered an essential part of menopause care to look after the health of bones by giving oestrogen replacement, usually as HRT and sometimes as the pill (combined oral contraceptive); see Chapter 5 for more.

The evidence is that HRT will help prevent bone loss, however old you are, and that the benefits will continue while you stay on it. This benefit has to be weighed up against potential risks associated with HRT, especially as you get older, and there may be a time when, on balance, HRT is not the best choice just for your bones. As you approach 60 years and beyond, you may want to discuss whether it is appropriate to stay on HRT for this reason or if other medical options are suitable.

Other ways of looking after your bones are discussed in Chapter 2.

Heart health

I did not realise that women were at risk of heart disease – I thought it was mainly a man's problem.

I had no idea that HRT was protecting my heart when I went on it at 50.

There has been a lot of controversy as to whether HRT is good for the heart or is harmful. Early studies indicated that it was good, but then a large study in the US suggested it was not and that it might even be harmful. Since then, more studies have broken the data down more carefully and have looked at whether it makes a difference how old you are when you start HRT, and how long it is since you went through menopause. Current research suggests that if you use HRT as a young woman with early menopause, it is beneficial to the heart. If you have no pre-existing heart problems and start HRT under the age of 60 or within ten years of your periods stopping, it is not harmful and may indeed be beneficial.

What is in HRT?

Oestrogen

After the menopause, oestrogen levels fall (you do not need a blood test to confirm this), and it is this lack that HRT aims to replace. Doses of HRT aim to give back enough oestrogen to alleviate symptoms and in a way that sustains an even oestrogen level in your body rather than the irregular levels that occur during the peri-menopause and soon after.

Oestrogens used in HRT are described as 'natural' rather than 'synthetic'. This means that they closely mimic the oestrogen produced by your body before menopause. This makes them different from the contraceptive pill, which uses synthetic oestrogen. There are two basic types of oestrogen used in HRT for menopausal symptoms:

- Oestradiol – the type which is closest to your own oestrogen; and
- Conjugated oestrogens – a mix of oestrogens, still described as 'natural' but not as close to your own oestrogen.

Oestrogen therapy aims to make you feel better, to lessen symptoms or, better still, eliminate them entirely. The right HRT for you makes you feel normal again, with few or no menopausal symptoms and hopefully no side effects. Oestrogen can be prescribed in different doses and may be given to you in various ways, e.g. tablets, patches or gels. Your doctor will ask you about the severity of your symptoms and decide which dose might be best for you based on that and on your age – younger women may need slightly higher doses in order to feel well. If you have been on HRT for a while, your doctor might suggest reducing the oestrogen dose and then perhaps stopping it altogether. If your symptoms are mainly vaginal – soreness, dryness or painful sex, you will be advised to use vaginal oestrogen, which is quite different to other types of HRT (see later in this chapter). Before prescribing HRT your doctor or nurse will ask a few questions to make sure that it is suitable for you and to rule out any medical reasons for not using it (see – 'Who should not use HRT?', below). If you have had a hysterectomy, for example, then you use 'oestrogen only' HRT. If you still have your womb, you need 'combined HRT' and you will be offered HRT that contains progestogen as well as oestrogen. These two hormones may be combined into one convenient tablet or patch or may be 'tailor-made' using separate medicines.

Progestogen/progesterone

It will help to explain the terms used, as it can be confusing:

◆ **Progesterone** – a hormone naturally produced by the body.

◆ **Progestogen** – synthetically produced to have progesterone-like effects on the body. There are different types of these, and many are used in HRT.

◆ **Micronised progesterone** – synthetically produced, to closely mimic progesterone, and similar to a body's own progesterone in terms of molecular structure. This is sometimes used in HRT and may be described as 'natural progesterone' because it is close to your own hormones in make-up and in how it works.

In this section, whenever the word 'progestogen' is used, it could equally be micronised progesterone that is being referred to, depending on the HRT combination you use.

If you have not had a hysterectomy and need HRT, a type of HRT will be prescribed that contains both oestrogen and progestogen/progesterone. Progestogen is similar to the body's hormone progesterone, and is needed to ensure the safety of oestrogen to the womb. Oestrogen, both in a natural cycle before menopause and with HRT afterwards, causes the lining of the womb (called the endometrium), to thicken. In a natural cycle, before menopause, the monthly period stops this from building up over time. Oestrogen in HRT will gradually lead to a thickening of the womb lining unless progestogen is also given alongside it, often in the same tablet or patch. Progestogen helps keep the womb lining healthy and is essential if you have a womb and want HRT. If you still have your womb and inadvertently use oestrogen-only HRT, also called 'unopposed oestrogen', there is a risk that the womb lining might start to develop unhealthy cells that could potentially be harmful if left untreated. By using combined oestrogen and progestogen HRT, you prevent this from happening. Instead of progestogen, some HRT uses micronised progesterone. This still protects the womb, and it is thought that it may have fewer side effects and perhaps presents less risk for some women (see the section on the risks of HRT, later in this chapter).

Progestogen releasing Intra-Uterine System (IUS or coil)

The coil containing progestogen (Mirena) is commonly used for long-acting contraception. If you are starting HRT with one of these already in place, you can use it as the progestogen part of your HRT, as long as it has not been in for longer than five years. If you had the Mirena put in as contraception or for heavy periods more than five years ago, it would need changing before you can use it as HRT. This is discussed further, under contraception, in Chapter 2.

Cyclical or continuous?

The role of progestogen or progesterone in HRT is to protect the endometrium (womb lining) and to ensure the safety of the oestrogen alongside it. The way that the progestogen part is given will vary according to how close you are to menopause when you start HRT.

Peri-menopausal or within a year of stopping periods?

I started to get my symptoms even though I had not had any change in my periods.

I did not realise that starting HRT might mean having regular periods again.

If you are still having periods and want to start HRT, or if you have missed a few but not yet gone twelve months without a period, you will be prescribed 'cyclical' or 'sequential' HRT. This means that every day, alongside the oestrogen, you also use some progestogen, but only for part of the month. Usually, it is incorporated into the patch or tablet you are using, so that you may notice a different-coloured tablet or a change in the patch after around two weeks, although no differences might be noticeable at all. This type of HRT generally results in a short monthly bleed that is not usually heavy. You would expect to get this bleed towards the end of the HRT packet or just into the new one. There is no break between packets with any HRT. If you are still using this HRT at around the age of 54, or sometimes after five years or so of HRT, you may be switched to continuous, or 'bleed-free' HRT. It is thought to be better for the womb lining if you make this switch when staying on HRT, but if you prefer to continue monthly bleeds you can discuss this.

Not had a natural period for a year or more?

I really hoped they would go, but I still have flushes even though my periods stopped a while ago.

If you start HRT more than one year after natural periods stop, you will be prescribed continuous HRT. This means that each tablet or patch has a bit of both oestrogen and progestogen in them and will be the same colour and type throughout the packet. The aim of this treatment is to be 'bleed-free', that is for you not to have a monthly bleed. Sometimes you can get some light bleeding at the beginning of this treatment, but

Summary of how HRT is given

Your circumstances	How you will take HRT
Hysterectomy	Oestrogen only
Mirena (IUS) inserted in last five years	Oestrogen (along with progestogen from your IUS)
Periods not yet stopped, period in the last twelve months?	Oestrogen with cyclical progestogen or progesterone, usually resulting in a monthly bleed
Periods stopped. No period for twelve months or more?	Oestrogen with continuous progestogen/progesterone. Aims to be period-free after an initial settling-in phase

this usually settles by three months to no bleeding at all. If bleeding continues beyond that, you may need a change in dose or type of HRT.

> **Recommendation**
> If you are still seeing some bleeding after six months on continuous HRT, you should report it to your doctor.

For some women, HRT might include testosterone, alongside oestrogen (and progestogen if needed). Often this will be for young women and in this book I discuss it in Chapter 5.

How is HRT given?

There are various forms of HRT and, for many women, it will be your choice which you use. Your prescriber might suggest one type over another, and there may be medical reasons why one might suit you more, but often it is a personal choice. Factors to consider if you are choosing:

◆ How easy is it to remember daily tablets?
◆ Can you physically swallow tablets with ease?
◆ Would you mind the physical reminder of the patch on your skin (usually on the bottom) or would that upset you?

- Is there any reason that you usually avoid tablets, e.g., allergies, stomach problems?
- What contraception are you using? Could that be combined with an HRT?
- Would you prefer to avoid tablets and therefore choose patch or gel?
- Do you only need vaginal oestrogen (for vaginal symptoms) and so could avoid other types?

Tablets

I chose tablets for convenience. I find them easy to remember and no hassle.

Tablets are easy to take, convenient, and come in all sorts of doses and types of HRT. This gives you the advantage of being able to switch doses easily or try different tablets with slightly different hormones in them if one does not agree with you. You can take tablets whether you still have periods, recently missed a period or have not had one for a while – there will be one to suit you whatever stage of menopause you are at. You can also easily change from cyclical to continuous HRT tablets when the time comes.

If you have no medical conditions, are of average weight for your height and don't smoke, you can consider tablets if you want and may in fact be offered them first if you do not express a preference.

Tips for using HRT tablets:

- It does not matter if you take them in the morning

or at night, but try to stick to around the same time every day.

◆ If you miss one, take it later the same day, but not two together.

◆ If you regularly forget tablets, you might see some spotting.

◆ You can take HRT tablets at the same time as most other tablets.

◆ Always start with the first tablet in the pack and work your way through in the right order.

Patches

I chose patches as I thought they would be easier to remember than daily tablets.

I was recommended patches because I am overweight.

I was surprised at how well they stick.

HRT patches are usually positioned on the round part of your bottom or tummy area and changed either once or twice a week, depending on the brand. The average-dose patches are generally around the size of a 50p piece or smaller, and they get bigger as doses increase. They usually stick well and can be worn in the shower or swimming pool. You may find that one patch brand sticks better than another, so you may need to try a couple of types if you find them coming unstuck. If they do come unstuck, they will not work properly as the hormone will not absorb across the skin effectively.

Patches are available as both oestrogen-only patches or combined oestrogen/progestogen patches, so you can use them whether you have had a hysterectomy or not. They come in both cyclical or continuous types of HRT so are suitable at whatever stage of menopause you are at.

Tips for using patches:

◆ To use the patch, remove the backing paper and try not to touch the sticky area too much before applying to dry skin.

◆ Do not apply to broken skin, e.g. psoriasis or eczema-affected skin.

◆ You may see small black sticky rings where the patch has been (like when removing a plaster): baby oil will easily remove this.

◆ When changing patches, use a slightly different area of skin.

◆ Remember to remove the old one when putting a new one on!

Gels

I like the gel because it is invisible to others.

I have sensitive skin, but the gel is just fine.

In the UK, there are two types of gels available for HRT: one in a pump pack with measured doses, a bit like a large toothpaste dispenser; and one that comes with each dose in an individual sachet. Gels are not available with progestogen, so are not suitable to be used alone by women who have not had a hysterectomy. If you still have a womb and want to use HRT gel, you will also need to be prescribed a progestogen or progesterone alongside it. Some women use gel alongside a progestogen-containing intrauterine system (Mirena coil), which is a convenient way of taking progestogen if you do not mind the coil and it has been changed within the last five years. Gels are usually applied to upper outer arms or outer thighs and are applied as a thin layer of gel and then allowed to dry. Do not rub the gel away completely. It takes a few minutes to dry and should be applied to dry, unmoisturised skin. Once the gel has fully dried, which only takes a few minutes, you can use creams and so on.

Tips for using gels:

◆ Remember to give the gel time to dry before applying creams or getting dressed.

◆ You can use sun lotion on the area you apply gel to but wait until after the gel has fully dried.

◆ Once the gel has dried it will not be transferred on to anyone else.

◆ Wash your hands after applying the gel so that it is not transferred to anyone else, e.g. children, partners or pets.

◆ Do not use the gels internally, including the vagina.

Advantages of patches and gels

Both patches and gels are described as 'transdermal

HRT', meaning 'through the skin'. Avoiding taking hormones in tablet form has some advantages for some women:

◆ It avoids the chance of nausea associated with tablets for some women.

◆ It has a lesser effect on thrombosis (blood clotting) – important if your personal risk is considered to be higher than average.

◆ There is less chance of triggering migraine, in women who have them, as the hormones release gradually.

◆ They are better for women with absorption difficulties, e.g., with Crohn's disease or other gastrointestinal upsets.

◆ There is lesser risk of stroke than with tablets (although the risk with tablets is small for most women).

◆ Most are similar to your own oestrogen so they feel 'natural'.

When discussing types of HRT, you may be recommended patches or gels in order to minimise the risk of venous thrombosis (blood clots), a small risk with tablets. This would particularly be the case if you are assessed to have a slightly higher than average background risk of thrombosis and might include:

◆ If you are overweight

◆ If you smoke

◆ If you have someone in your close family who has had stroke or thrombosis

◆ If you had a thrombosis many years ago.

You might also be offered them if you have health conditions such as:

◆ High blood pressure controlled with medication
◆ Diabetes
◆ Migraine
◆ Epilepsy
◆ Crohn's disease.

Both tablets and patches should be effective in relieving symptoms, if the dose is right for you. You may need to try one or the other before finding the one that suits you best.

Bioidenticals

The term 'bioidentical' simply means the same molecular make-up as that produced by your body. Many HRTs could be described in this way. Oestradiol is bioidentical oestrogen, and micronised progesterone is bioidentical progesterone. So if you want this type of HRT, it is available on the NHS as conventional HRT.

You may see 'bioidentical HRT' advertised that claims to individually prepare a formulation of hormones that is right just for you, based on salivary hormone tests. This may seem attractive but note that, at present, the Medicines and Healthcare products Regulatory Agency (MHRA), the body in the UK that oversees the safety of medicines, does not regulate these formulations or review their safety. Unlike conventional HRT, doses and purity will vary, and risks are currently unknown.

Vaginal oestrogen

My menopausal symptoms are gone but I still have this dryness and sex is painful.

I feel dry, itchy and uncomfortable in my vaginal area. It's not just about sex, it is all the time.

Sometimes called 'vaginal HRT', this type of treatment is just for relief of vaginal symptoms. It is poorly absorbed into the body so will not treat general menopausal symptoms at all. For this reason, you may be able to use it even if you cannot use general HRT. You may need vaginal oestrogen alongside other HRT if your vaginal symptoms are particularly troublesome, and you can continue it even after you stop general HRT. If you use vaginal oestrogen at the recommended doses you will not need to use a progestogen as well and you do not need any particular tests before using it.

Vaginal symptoms, along with mild bladder symptoms like frequency (going more often), nocturia (waking at night to pee), and urgency (when you gotta go, you gotta go!), will respond well to vaginal oestrogen as long as you keep using it. If you stop, the symptoms will eventually return, so short-term treatments will not be very useful.

You may be offered one of three different ways of using vaginal oestrogen: all will be effective so you should be offered a choice. Go for the one that appeals to you and that you will be willing to use:

◆ **Vaginal tablets** – a tiny tablet, on the end of an

applicator, is inserted into the vagina like a tampon, and the tablet pops out and sticks to the top of the vagina, slowly releasing oestrogen. You throw the applicator away. After an initial two-week nightly dose, you use the tablets twice weekly.

Advantage – feels dry, slim, new applicator each time.

Disadvantage – no moistness on application, applicator quite long.

◆ **Cream** – you fill an applicator with cream and insert vaginally, pushing the cream through the applicator. Again, follow a nightly dose for two weeks then apply twice weekly.

Advantage – feels moisturising, applicator easy to use.

Disadvantage – reusable applicator has to be washed, some find the product messy.

◆ **Ring** – a small ring is inserted by you high into the vagina. This stays in place for three months and slowly releases oestrogen. It can remain in during sex, although some women prefer to remove it and put it back later.

Advantage – long-acting, feels dry, cannot be felt when in place.

Disadvantage – inserted with fingers, stays in the vagina (high up).

Vaginal lubricants and moisturisers were discussed in Chapter 3. You may find that you need this as well as vaginal oestrogen. The oestrogen is a treatment for lack of oestrogen and addresses the underlying cause of the dryness or soreness, while the lubricants, in particular, will ensure comfort during sex.

> **Recommendation**
>
> If you have unexpected bleeding while using vaginal oestrogen, report it to your doctor.

Side effects and risks of HRT

I definitely want to think about this. I want to be responsible.

I understand the risk now and can balance that against the benefits, to me, of feeling back to normal.

I know that any medication carries risks and side effects, HRT is no different.

Guidance from NICE (National Institute for Health and Care Excellence) says that for women with symptoms, the risks of HRT are small and usually outweighed by the benefits. The full link to the NICE Guidance, which has information for doctors and for women, is available in the Resources chapter. You will be most interested in your own personal risks and that is why you need a full and individual discussion about HRT before starting it. You will want to ask:

◆ What are the known risks of HRT; and
◆ How do these risks apply to me?

Before starting HRT, as well as understanding the

known risks with its use, you will want to know about possible side effects that you may experience. As with any medicine, these need to be balanced against the benefits you will get from being on the treatment. For most women, starting HRT around the age of natural menopause or for early menopause, HRT will be low risk, but only you can decide whether any risk, however small, is worth taking in order to treat your symptoms.

Venous thrombosis (also called deep vein thrombosis, DVT)

Venous thrombosis is the term that describes the formation of blood clots in deep veins of the body, usually the legs. It causes pain and swelling and can lead to serious medical complications. Such thrombosis can affect anyone, and there are factors that increase the chance of you getting one, including:

◆ Having a family history of blood clots
◆ Prolonged inactivity, e.g., after an operation, or on a long journey if you do not move much
◆ Having already had a blood clot
◆ Having a medical condition that may cause your blood to thicken more quickly
◆ Pregnancy
◆ Being overweight.

Taking HRT by tablet very slightly increases the risk of thrombosis. There is no increased risk of blood clots from patches or gels. It's estimated that for every 1,000 women taking HRT tablets for seven and a half years, fewer than two will develop a blood clot (NICE Guidance 2015). In statistical terms, this is considered a 'small' risk. To put it into perspective, that is lower than your risk during pregnancy.

If you have risk factors for blood clots, like those above, you are likely to be advised to use patches or gels as a first choice.

Heart (cardiovascular) disease and stroke

Cardiovascular disease is a term used to describe conditions that affect the heart or blood vessels. It encompasses conditions like angina and heart attacks as well as stroke and arterial disease, which cause impaired circulation. We know there are certain factors, called risk factors, that may suggest you are at a higher risk for heart disease and these are discussed in Chapter 2.

NICE Guidance, after review of the scientific evidence, states that:

1. HRT does not significantly increase the risk of cardiovascular disease when started before 60 years of age.

2. Oestrogen-only HRT is associated with no or reduced risk of heart disease and combined HRT (i.e. oestrogen and progestogen) is associated with little or no increase in risk of heart disease.

3. Oestrogen tablets but not patches are associated with a small increase in the risk of stroke, although the

normal risk of women under 60 having a stroke is low, so the overall risk is small.

NICE Guidance did not review the data for women starting HRT after the age of 60, and if this applies to you, you will need a careful risk assessment and discussion before starting HRT. You may need to be seen by a specialist, who can help you decide if the benefits outweigh the potential risk. This will depend on your general health and your medical and family history, as well as the type and dose of HRT you are given.

Breast cancer

Once I understood the risk, I felt more confident using HRT.

It was probably my fear of breast cancer that stopped me taking HRT.

This is probably the one that worries women the most because we all know someone who has had breast cancer or who knows someone who did. At around 50 you will be invited to participate in the national breast screening programme where you will undergo those mammograms that squeeze and press so hard on your breasts. See Chapter 2 for information about cancer screening.

For many years, it has been known that some types of HRT may increase the risk of breast cancer when used for more than five years, and recently it has become clearer through research that if so, the small risk is with combined HRT rather than with HRT that contains only oestrogen. This does not mean that you can take oestrogen-only HRT, however, unless you have had a hysterectomy. The progestogen or progesterone part of HRT is essential to the safety of your womb.

A small increase in breast cancer risk is linked to long-term use of combined HRT, probably starting to rise after five years or so of HRT and as you stay on HRT for ten or fifteen years after the natural age of menopause (around 50). If you start HRT much younger than this, it is not thought to increase your risk of breast cancer above your usual risk, because your ovaries would normally have been doing the same job, had they been working properly. This is particularly important for young women who may need to use HRT for many years to take them to 50.

Breast cancer is common, and some women will get it whether or not they are on HRT – this is called the 'background risk' or 'population risk'. This means that some women may still get breast cancer on HRT. In this instance, it is not the HRT that has necessarily led to cancer but the background risk continuing despite starting HRT.

I did not know that other factors, like being overweight or drinking a couple of glasses of wine a night, increased my breast cancer risk by a similar amount to taking HRT.

Other factors in life also increase your individual risk of breast cancer (see Chapter 2). This includes being overweight, smoking, daily alcohol, little or no exercise and a diet high in saturated fats. In fact, the risk with long-term combined HRT is probably equivalent to being overweight or drinking two glasses of wine a day.

This is important, of course, and you may choose to limit this risk, but it is not as great a risk as you might sometimes think reading the media coverage on HRT.

If you have women in your close family, such as your mother or sister, who have had breast cancer, you will want to think carefully about whether the background risk for you is higher. It may be, too, that men in the family have had prostate or bowel cancer – this might suggest a family link with the disease. If this is the case, you may still be able to take HRT after a discussion about your personal risks.

Most women after the age of 50 do not need HRT for longer than five years; you are more likely to use it for a short period to get through a difficult time, say a year or two, when the breast cancer risks are at their lowest. Some do stay on HRT for much longer, and if this is you, you will need to balance the small possible risks of staying on against the disadvantages of stopping. Different women will make different decisions, which is again why it is so important that you get the individualised menopause care that health professionals advocate.

Ovarian cancer

Ovarian cancer is rare. A link with ovarian cancer and HRT is not clear, with the evidence conflicting. If there is a risk, it appears to be very small and only occurs after long-term use of HRT. Again, if someone close to you has had ovarian cancer it will be of more significance, and you may want to seek specialist advice before using HRT.

Womb cancer (endometrial cancer)

We have discussed the importance of progestogen or progesterone as part of HRT if you still have a womb. This is because it has been known for many years that oestrogen on its own, in women with a womb, can lead to an 'overgrowth' of the womb lining. This can lead to irregular bleeding, which is a nuisance, but more importantly it could result in unhealthy cell changes in the womb lining, which, if left untreated, might turn cancerous.

Each type of HRT, cyclical or continuous, has been formulated to ensure that your womb lining has the necessary progestogen protection in order to prevent this overgrowth. This means that HRT does not increase the risk of endometrial cancer when used correctly.

Recommendation

If your bleeding pattern on HRT changes from what is normal for you, you should report it to your doctor.

Side effects

My breasts felt sore for a couple of weeks, but it settled down.

I knew I had started something, but soon got used to it.

I felt my side effects went on too long, so I asked my doctor for a lower dose, which suited me more.

I had to try three different HRTs before I found one that suited me.

Any medicine can cause side effects, and HRT is no different. Fortunately, with HRT they are usually short-lived, settling down within about a month or so as your body adjusts to the hormone changes. Common side effects in the early days are due to the oestrogen and include:

◆ Breast tenderness or heaviness
◆ Nipple sensitivity
◆ Slight nausea
◆ Leg cramps.

If side effects such as these continue beyond a couple of months, you might want to discuss reducing the dose or changing the type of HRT, or perhaps the way you take it – e.g., from tablets to patches / gels.

Sometimes it can be the progestogen you use that contributes to side effects, and if that is the case they may sometimes continue longer term if you do not switch treatments. HRTs have a variety of different progestogens and sometimes a different type will suit you better, or you may try an HRT regimen using micronised progesterone. There is one type of HRT in the UK which avoids the use of progestogen altogether and has a different hormonal component to protect the womb lining, useful mainly in women who have tried all the various progestogen combinations first.

How do you know you are on the right HRT?

I tried about three before I began to forget I was on it and just felt normal.

It is quite common to try more than one HRT before finding one that suits you. HRT comes in a whole variety of different doses, types and routes of delivery, so, with each woman having individual needs, it sometimes needs 'tweaking' to find the one that suits you best. I am often asked, 'what is the best HRT?' and that is difficult to answer as what is 'best' for you may not be 'best' for someone else. The right HRT for you is the one that is the right dose to make you feel normal, the right type (for example if you have medical conditions that suggest a particular type of HRT), and in the right combination of oestrogen and progestogen. In any case, it is wise to keep the dose as low as you need (some will need higher doses than others) and to only use it for the time that you need it, which might be a few months for some women and many years for others.

Who should not use HRT?

My doctor told me I could not use HRT, but I am not sure why.

When I speak with women, I discover that many are told that they cannot use HRT when in fact there is no apparent medical reason for this. It may be because some healthcare professionals are not confident about prescribing HRT or are unsure about women with certain medical conditions using it. Quite rightly, they prescribe only within the area in which they are competent and confident, but this occasionally leaves women unsupported or without adequate explanation. Chapter 8 has ideas for approaching your doctor, getting the best from your consultation, and suggestions of other ways to access HRT, as well as via your GP.

You will not usually be prescribed HRT if:

- You have had cancer that might be influenced by hormones, e.g., breast or womb.
- You have recently had a heart attack, a blood clot (thrombosis) or stroke.
- You have unusually heavy, prolonged or frequent periods (this needs checking out before using HRT).
- Something is wrong with your liver – liver disease.

There are some medical conditions that mean that, although you can use HRT, some caution is required before you take it. It may mean using a particular type or dose or extra monitoring when on it. Below are some of the conditions that may affect your use of HRT.

Fibroids

Fibroids are non-cancerous growths that occur in the womb, sometimes leading to heavy bleeding and pain. If you have a scan of the womb for something else, small fibroids might be detected that you were unaware of because they gave you no problems. HRT will not usually have any effect on small fibroids and these usually shrink of their own accord after menopause. If you have large fibroids that have caused heavy bleeding and you go onto HRT while still having periods, you may find that the fibroids do not shrink and continue to cause bleeding problems. Changing the type of HRT and monitoring the fibroids when you first start HRT can usually resolve this.

Endometriosis

Endometriosis occurs when tissue outside the womb starts to behave like the lining of the womb. So whenever you have a period, this tissue also prepares to bleed, sometimes leading to pain. Commonly this tissue may be around the tubes and ovaries or near the bowel. After the menopause, endometriosis usually shrinks and seldom causes more problems. If you go onto cyclical HRT and still have endometrial deposits (tissue), this tissue may bleed like normal womb lining, reactivating your endometriosis pain. This is less likely to happen if you have a few months of no periods before stopping HRT (when the deposits will have shrunk) or if you wait until you have had no periods for a year and can go on continuous HRT, which is less likely to stimulate the deposits. If you have had surgery for endometriosis you may be recommended to use combined HRT for a while, even if you have had a hysterectomy, again to ensure that any deposits are not activated.

Epilepsy

You can take HRT with epilepsy. You may be

recommended patches or gel to try to ensure a steady absorption of hormones and in order to make sure that there is no interaction with your epilepsy medication.

Migraine

You can take HRT with migraine. If you take HRT for other menopausal symptoms, for example flushes, HRT may aggravate your migraines, may improve them, and will sometimes make no difference. Unlike advice for the contraceptive pill, you do not have to avoid HRT because you have migraines, but you will be recommended to have patches or gels (with progestogen/ progesterone if needed). This will help avoid hormonal fluctuations that, for some women, worsen migraine. If you have migraine with aura, and want HRT, you will be advised to use patches or gels. Many migraines are unrelated to hormones and HRT will have no effect on these.

High blood pressure (hypertension)

High blood pressure puts pressure on the heart and blood vessels and, if left untreated, can lead to health problems such as an increased risk of heart attack or stroke. You may not know you have high blood pressure unless you have had it measured. HRT does not influence blood pressure significantly so you can use it even if you are being treated for high blood pressure. If you are using HRT and develop high blood pressure, the blood pressure will need monitoring and treating in the same way that it would if you were not on HRT. If you want HRT alongside blood pressure treatment, you may be recommended patches and gels before tablets.

How to decide whether to use HRT

You may be recommended HRT, or you may be thinking about it yourself. Here are some questions you might want to consider to help you make that decision. Thinking through these questions will help to equip you for that medical consultation when you ask about HRT.

1. Have you had the menopause early, before the age of 45? If so, you are likely to be recommended HRT.

2. Will HRT help? Menopausal symptoms will improve, but you may still have to address other issues like stress, overwork, relationship problems and other health concerns.

3. What are your personal risks with HRT? This means taking into account your medical history and that of close family.

4. Can you address your symptoms in other ways? How much do they bother you?

5. Which type of HRT will you need? Have you had a hysterectomy; have your periods stopped yet? If not, do you mind the return of a monthly bleed?

6. How long might you use it? Most women use HRT to see them through the short-term symptoms of menopause. For some this might be more than five years, and no one can tell you how long your symptoms will last.

Is it ever too late to start HRT?

I have put up with symptoms for so long, have I left it too late?

Most women who use HRT do so sometime in the decade between 50 and 60 years. It is unusual to start HRT after the age of around 60 or later than ten years after your periods have stopped because cardiovascular risks might be increased for you (unless you are young). However, it does depend on your personal health: we all know that not all 60-year-olds are the same, and that some are very fit, have taken care to exercise, don't smoke and are fortunate not to have any medical conditions. If you are over 60 or have existing heart problems and want to start HRT, you will need a careful assessment of risk. This might include considering:

◆ Do you smoke?
◆ Are you overweight?
◆ Do you exercise?
◆ Do you know your cholesterol levels?
◆ Is there a family history of heart attacks under 60?

Whether or not you can start HRT over the age of 60 will depend on individual assessment: in other words, your personal risks and how much you need HRT – i.e. how bad your symptoms are. Can you reduce your risk, perhaps by stopping smoking or losing weight if HRT is needed? In any case, if your symptoms are predominantly vaginal, you can use vaginal oestrogen at any age (see vaginal treatments later in this chapter).

> ### Recommendation
> If you are over 60 or if it is more than ten years since your periods stopped and you still have symptoms, you may be able to use HRT: discuss with your doctor.

Do you need any health checks before starting HRT?

I was surprised how quickly I was prescribed it. I thought there would be more tests.

The most important health check will be of your general health and other medical conditions. That will influence whether HRT can be prescribed and the type of HRT that will be best for you. If you have any medical conditions, they may influence the type of HRT you can use, or whether it is appropriate for you.

Your blood pressure will be checked and, if high, it may need to be monitored for a short while before starting HRT. If it's high and regulated with medication, HRT may be started, usually as patches or gels.

Your body mass index, which is calculated by your height and weight, will influence the type of HRT suggested for you. If you are quite overweight, patches and gels will be recommended first.

> **Recommendation**
>
> If you see anyone other than your GP for HRT,
> remember that they will not have your medical history
> to hand, so you will need to tell them yourself.

Coming off HRT?

Going on HRT was easy, coming off not quite so easy.

I felt so well on HRT, I was reluctant to come off: would I feel bad again?

It felt strange, just stopping HRT after so long on it. I chose to do so gradually, to give me confidence.

For some women, starting HRT is the easy decision, but deciding when and how to stop can be harder. You may think: 'Am I just postponing the inevitable? Will all my symptoms come back?' HRT does not postpone your symptoms, which is reassuring. No one knows how long you were destined to have symptoms for, but, let's say five years. If you stay on HRT for three years, when you stop, your symptoms will still be there, but if you stay on five years, they may not. So sometimes if you stop HRT, your symptoms do come back, and you might decide to stay on a bit longer and come off again in six to twelve months.

If you are on a higher dose of HRT, it makes sense to reduce the dose before stopping, and you may feel happier stopping gradually, rather than doing so suddenly. There is no harm in stopping HRT suddenly

– you may simply experience a few weeks of symptoms as your body adjusts. Speak to your prescriber to find out how best to tail off the particular HRT you are on – different ones are done in different ways.

Frequently asked questions about hormone replacement therapy (HRT)

1 *Who might want HRT?*

Any woman might consider the use of HRT. It may be because symptoms have become so bothersome that you are inclined to look for a solution. It could be that your menopause was early and you have been recommended HRT for health reasons until you reach the average age of menopause.

2 *How long do I take HRT?*

This is an individual choice. Some women use HRT for a few months or a couple of years to get through a difficult time, then they come off. Others use it for several years, because their symptoms seem to go on for a long time. Others use it for many years because they were young when the ovaries stopped working and they need the long-term health benefits.

3 *Do I have to have a bleed?*

If you have had a natural period in the last year, you will be given an HRT that usually results in a monthly bleed. For some, this is a disadvantage of starting HRT close to menopause. If you can wait until a year after your periods stop, you can take an HRT that leads to no bleeds (after a settling-in phase). Symptoms, though, are not always obliging enough to wait until that point, which is why women often start HRT earlier. If you have been on an HRT that produces a bleed for about five years, or if you reach the age of 54, you can often switch to a no-bleed HRT at that time.

4 *If I go on HRT, how will I know when I have gone through menopause?*

If you start HRT while still having periods, you will not know the actual time that you go through menopause. Does this matter? Not really, except to know when to stop using contraception, so the usual recommendation in this instance is to stop contraception at age 55.

5 *What are HRT implants?*

HRT implants (small pellets inserted under the skin, through a tiny cut), were popular some years ago, but the UK supplies have been withdrawn. Some specialist clinics can import supplies for existing users, but you are unlikely to be offered an implant as a new user now. Like all treatments, they came with advantages and disadvantages, and modern forms of HRT probably have more advantages.

6 *Does it matter if I take the HRT tablet at night or in the morning?*

Most HRT tablets can be taken at any time: just try to keep to roughly the same time each day in order to get into the habit and not miss pills. If you miss one, take it later in the day or next morning, but don't take two together to catch up – there is no need.

7 *Can I adjust my tablet-taking so as to push back my bleed when I go on holiday?*

Sometimes you can do this and if you want advice on how best to do it, ask your prescriber or pharmacist. Do not simply miss out parts of the packet as that could cause irregular bleeding in the long term. It is usually possible, with very minor tweaks to your HRT and only now and again, to change the bleed start, but doing this too often or unsupervised might cause problems so always check.

8 *If I start having periods again on HRT, does that make me fertile?*

No, HRT does not make your own ovaries work again and the bleeding does not indicate that you are fertile. If you start HRT while having periods, you will need to continue contraception for a time as your own ovaries may have intermittent activity alongside the HRT (see Chapter 2).

9 *Could I inadvertently take too much HRT? Would it be harmful if my dose was too high?*

If you take HRT as prescribed, you will not overdose. Doses are individual and some people need higher doses than others in order to control symptoms. If the dose seems a little high for you, your body will tell you, with side effects, such as breast tenderness, that continue beyond the initial few weeks settling-in period.

10 *Is it dangerous to just stop HRT – must I wean myself off gradually?*

It is not dangerous to simply stop HRT. Many women prefer to come off in a gradual fashion, first reducing the dose to the lowest, before finally stopping, as it makes them feel more in control and sometimes avoids possible 'rebound' symptoms, which might occur initially on stopping. It is your choice how to stop. If you take combined HRT, check with your prescriber if you want to gradually stop it.

11 *Reading this has made me realise that I am taking oestrogen-only HRT but I still have my womb. What should I do?*

If you have inadvertently been using an HRT that is not the most suitable, the first step is to see your GP to clarify the prescription. Sometimes computer errors creep in with similar-sounding HRT preparations (e.g. Evorel and Evorel Sequi) and mistakes might be missed. If you have a womb and used oestrogen-only HRT for more than three months, your doctor will suggest an ultrasound scan to check the womb lining. This will give an indication of the thickness of the womb lining and further treatment will be offered only if necessary. (It is often not needed, other than changing to a more appropriate HRT.)

12 *My GP says I have 'had my five years' of HRT but I don't want to come off. What can I do?*

There is no set length of time that you can be on HRT and, although your doctor is simply trying to minimise risk, this should be discussed with you so that you can make the choice. Risks will be individual to you and benefits will depend on why you are on HRT. Different women will make different choices. Ask your GP what the risks of staying on might be and say that you want to make an informed choice, given how well you feel on HRT. It may be time to review the way you take HRT and the dose you use too.

13 *Do I need to stop HRT before an operation?*

For a minor planned operation, not involving a long stay in hospital, you should not need to stop HRT. However, you should take time to discuss this several weeks in advance of the surgery and the final decision will lie with the surgeon and anaesthetist.

14 *I have been using HRT for nine weeks, but it does not seem to be working. Should I try a different one?*

By nine weeks, I would expect flushes and sweats to have lessened a bit, but you may not yet be getting maximum benefit. Other symptoms may take longer to improve with HRT. It is worth assessing again at twelve weeks. You may need a change in dose or type of HRT in order to achieve better symptom relief.

15 *I have been prescribed HRT, but when do I actually start it? It looks complicated.*

If you are still having periods, start the HRT near the beginning of a period, making sure that you start on tablet 1 of the packet. If your periods have stopped or you only see one occasionally, start as soon as you wish.

The next chapter is about women who are younger than normal when they suspect menopause and the particular considerations that are unique in this case. In Chapter 8, you will find information about how to access the right practitioner, what questions to ask, and how to be referred to a specialist for treatment if you need it.

chapter 5

Young menopause
Experiencing menopause if you are under 40

What's in a name?
Premature, early, or young menopause; premature ovarian failure or premature ovarian insufficiency

Although menopause can happen at any age, for women there is a time of life when it is expected, a time that you have prepared for psychologically and when it comes as no surprise, even if the journey through it might be a bit rocky. At 50, you know it is going to happen. To the woman under the age of 40, it usually comes as a surprise, or even a shock. Even if, in the back of your mind, you were wondering if what was happening was the menopause, you will have hoped it was something else. 'Maybe it's stress; or perhaps I am overworking; or is it my diet?' All of this has probably gone through your mind before contemplating a diagnosis of early menopause. In fact, it is possible that you did not even consider such a diagnosis; after all, you may be thinking, women don't become menopausal that young, do they? Even getting the diagnosis can take a few months, or even more, of investigations. Some clinicians consider it such an unusual occurrence that patients are persuaded to wait several months before starting tests, and others are given nothing but reassurance. All this time, you face uncertainties about the future. Will you get pregnant? Will your hormones come back to normal? What is happening and what can be done about it? To be fair, diagnosis is not always simple, and it may be that several weeks, or even months, of tests will be needed before a definite diagnosis can be made. Because of the profound implications, both physically and psychologically, this is not a diagnosis that anyone wants to make without absolute certainty, so tests will need to be repeated over time in order to build a clear picture of what is happening with your hormones. To complicate matters, you may be experiencing inter-mittent hormonal activity for some time before finally reaching a stage that could be described as 'ovarian insufficiency'. So you need a combination of patience and perseverance with your clinician to ensure that tests are completed in a timely but appropriate manner.

Won't I get symptoms?

It wasn't the symptoms that took me to the doctor, it was worry about a lack of periods every so often, which just didn't seem right.

You might think that menopausal symptoms will give it away, but young women do not always get the classic symptoms of hot flushes and night sweats. Some may not notice symptoms like tiredness, reduced sex drive and mood swings until they are offered treatment, and then suddenly realise quite how much better they feel. The onset of menopausal changes can be gradual and can fluctuate, so you may get times when you feel fine and other times when you get symptoms. This is a normal part of the transition into menopause at any age and particularly if you are young.

Which name is correct?

The language used to describe early menopause varies, both among women and among health professionals. Professionals prefer the term 'premature ovarian insufficiency' to be used in women whose ovaries cease to function effectively under 40 years of age, even if you still see occasional periods. This term accurately reflects the fact that your ovaries are not working properly but that you might be in a state of flux, which will eventually lead to 'menopause'. It can sometimes take several months or even years to go from the beginning of ovarian insufficiency, when you might get symptoms, or start having difficulties conceiving, to complete menopause, which simply means the absolute last menstrual period. Some women have occasional periods on and off, yet would still be described as having 'ovarian insufficiency'. Others clearly stop their periods early on in the process and never have another. Either way, blood tests will confirm the diagnosis but, because hormones fluctuate so much, it can take several tests to confirm it. The term 'menopause' is used by women of all ages to describe the time of hormonal transition but strictly speaking simply refers to the actual last period (see Chapter 1).

If you go through menopausal changes under the age of 40, it is usually described as 'premature'. This is a medical definition and is used worldwide by health professionals to try to classify ages of menopause from a medical point of view. If you are 40 to 45 years of age, you may not be described as having menopause 'prematurely', but it would still be considered early and is often described as such ('early menopause'): around 5 per cent of women under 45 years of age go through menopause early. Whether your menopause is defined medically as 'premature' or 'early' makes little difference to you personally, as the effects are the same and the treatment and support the same too. From a medical perspective, it is those under 40 who are considered to need most hormonal support because of the long-term health implications which will be discussed later. Occasionally young women cannot use hormone therapy after early menopause and this is discussed more in Chapter 4.

You will find that in this book the terms 'premature ovarian insufficiency' and 'early menopause' are used interchangeably as most of the advice will fit all groups of young women, whether their menopause is natural or surgical and whether they are under 40 or under 45 years of age.

'Surgical menopause' is used when the ovaries have been removed by an operation. Ovaries are responsible for hormonal production so removing them causes immediate menopause, without any doubt and with all the consequences starting straightaway. For example, menopause symptoms, such as flushes and sweats, can occur very soon after surgery. Usually, such surgery is planned ahead of time, so you should have had the opportunity to ask questions and make a plan for ongoing treatment if suitable. If it is recommended that you have your ovaries removed by operation, find out if you will be recommended hormone treatment afterwards and when you might be able to start it, and discuss the types that are available to you (see Chapter 4 for information on HRT and Chapter 6 for information about menopause or HRT after cancer).

The term 'premature menopause' is generally avoided unless surgically induced. This is because using the word 'menopause' implies finality whereas many women have a gradual ovarian decline, with occasional episodes of ovarian function occurring during a time of hormonal turmoil, and this leads to difficulty with diagnosis and management. This will be discussed more later.

Why it happens

The worst part for me was just not being able to explain to my loved ones, my partner, my mum ... why this has happened. They wanted reasons and there weren't any. That made it very hard for us all to accept.

Premature ovarian insufficiency (POI) is not rare, with around 1 in 100 women under the age of 40 experiencing it, and 1 in 1,000 under 30. It is less common in the teens and twenties but it does happen, and no woman is too young for the diagnosis. Although it is not rare, it is quite possible that you will not have knowingly met anyone else with it. It is not something that women often share with anyone other than close family or loved ones and not something that comes up easily in conversation with friends unless you are very close. This can make it feel quite isolating and you may find it useful to seek support through networks such as Daisy Network, a support website for young women (details in the Resources section).

Premature ovarian insufficiency – spontaneous

I had been trying for a baby for a while, then the investigations indicated POI. Not only was I not going to have a baby, I was menopausal – so much to take in.

For many women, the first sign that there is a problem may be when you try to conceive. Investigation into fertility leads to a diagnosis of suspected ovarian insufficiency (POI). POI is not the only cause of infertility, though, so be reassured that, if pregnancy is your goal, many of the problems leading to infertility can be successfully treated. Other women notice an absence of periods, sometimes, but not always, accompanied by typical menopausal symptoms. Occasionally a medical cause can be found, but for many women no reason is identified.

Causes of premature ovarian insufficiency

◆ **Genetic** – any defect of the female sex chromosome can lead to ovarian failure. The most common form is Turner Syndrome, when early development of the ovary may be normal but the ovaries fail to mature and lead to puberty. Treatment usually starts as a child and continues long term to replace hormones that the body usually produces itself. Even small defects in the X chromosome can lead to early ovarian failure, often not detected until genetic testing is performed, perhaps because of family history of early menopause. At present, there is no treatment available to 'correct' these genes or chromosomes and research continues. Genetic testing may be suggested if menopause occurs under the age of 30 and if there is a family link of such young menopause. It is unusual to find a genetic cause, and there is a need for further research in this area.

◆ **Autoimmune conditions** – occasionally ovarian insufficiency is associated with conditions such as thyroid disease and adrenal disease, e.g. Addison's. The inflammation contributed by such conditions can also affect the ovaries. For this reason, it is common to test for autoantibodies early in the diagnosis process simply to rule out any other contributing factors that might be treatable.

◆ **External factors** – ovarian function can be interrupted by medical treatments such as chemotherapy or radiotherapy, by surgery close to the ovaries, and occasionally by an infection, such as sepsis.

It took me completely by surprise. I always assumed that whatever the problem with my lack of periods was, it would resolve. I was devastated to be told it was final.

Everything changed. I just wish I could wind back the clock and be normal.

If they could have at least given me a reason it happened, I would find it easier to cope with … it's hard wondering all the time if I caused it.

For many women, in fact, most women, no apparent cause is found, and it is described as 'idiopathic', which is very frustrating for women looking for a cause and then potentially a treatment. We all have such faith in the medical profession to 'put things right' that uncertainty is disarming and frustrating. Genuine premature ovarian failure cannot be corrected but there is a chance of hormonal activity leading right up to the final stages of ovarian insufficiency, so occasionally women appear to be in menopause and then ovarian activity starts again for a while before finally stopping altogether. This is why 'insufficiency' is the correct term rather than 'ovarian failure'. Counselling women is tricky because no one wants to give false hope that hormones may correct themselves, but women also need to know that spontaneous ovarian activity occasionally occurs. This is particularly important for women for whom pregnancy would not be good news since, very occasionally, surprises do happen, as hormonal activity in around 5 per cent of women may unexpectedly resume months or even years after the apparent loss of ovarian function.

Support and information

I tried so hard to find information aimed at my age – it was almost impossible.

Reading the leaflet was pretty depressing – made me feel old before my time.

I was very angry, with the diagnosis, with my future and with the lack of information.

Most resources and support materials are aimed at women going through menopause at the expected time, so pictures are of midlife women, and the general advice encompasses lifestyle and health issues relating to women in their fifties. Young women want and need tailored support, relevant and accurate for their needs. Daisy Network (www.daisynetwork.org.uk) is a particular resource aimed at young women going through menopause (or POI) and is a very useful place to look for specific advice and information .

Cancer charities such as Jo's Cervical Cancer Trust (https://jostrust.org.uk/) and Ovacome (http://www.ovacome.org.uk/) have specific information aimed at young women experiencing menopause as a result of cancer treatments. They also have stories from real women describing their transition into menopause through cancer treatment, which can be useful for others facing the same.

Surgical menopause

I did it [had risk-reducing oophorectomy] *for my*

*children, so they would not lose me like I lost my mum,
but now I have to cope with menopause – no one told me it
would be like this.*

Bilateral salpingo-oophorectomy (BSO), or removal of both ovaries and tubes, is not performed lightly in young women and may be the result of cancer treatment, severe endometriosis, severe premenstrual syndrome, cysts or infection. The surgery will have been considered essential, and menopause is an unwanted consequence of a very necessary treatment. Symptoms often occur quite soon after surgery, and if it is planned surgery it is helpful if options to manage symptoms have been discussed beforehand. Before the operation, take the time to speak to your consultant and ask specific questions, for example:

◆ Why is this surgery necessary, and is there an alternative?

◆ How will I feel afterwards – short and long term?

◆ How long is the usual recovery time?

◆ Will I be able to use hormone therapy afterwards and if so when should I start?

◆ What support will I be offered later if I need it? How do I access it?

If you carry a cancer genetic abnormality making ovarian or breast cancer a high possibility, you may be advised to consider surgical removal of ovaries, usually once your family is complete or by the age at which your family member had cancer. You may have family members who have had ovarian cancer, breast cancer or prostate cancer and been tested for the BRCA gene mutation after careful genetic counselling. This is called risk-reducing surgery and may be combined with breast surgery or long-term medication to reduce the risk of breast cancer or with increased breast surveillance using mammograms or magnetic resonance imaging (MRI).

You may have made the difficult choice to have a surgical menopause at a young age, in the knowledge that by doing so you greatly reduce your risk of cancer later on. Having your ovaries removed decreases that cancer risk. Ideally, you will have had an opportunity beforehand to discuss the impact that this will have both physically and psychologically, and the chance to put in place long-term plans for ensuring good health into the future, for example through promoting good bone health and preventing cardiovascular disease.

If you have risk-reducing BSO and have not had breast cancer you may be able to take HRT. A careful explanation as well as ongoing monitoring should be offered, either by the surgeon (gynaecologist) or by your own general practitioner. You should also be made aware that, if sexual problems arise following surgery, such as dryness or desire issues, help is available in the form of treatments and psychosexual support. NICE Guidance in the UK suggests that such women are seen by a healthcare professional with expertise in menopause, in order to discuss the options. You access such a specialist through your GP. It may help to do a little research yourself into specialist clinics and there is a basic list on the website www.menopausematters.co.uk (see Resources section). Not all specialists are on that list and your GP may know one locally that is not listed. Chapter 8 discusses how to access support and make the best of a consultation.

Induced menopause

Having cancer was awful, the treatments were awful, I was pleased to get through it all, then I faced menopause – double awful, just when I thought everything was over and I was 'getting my life back!'

Some women will receive treatments for cancer, which, while not surgically removing the ovaries, still cause them to become ineffective, leading to menopause. Some chemotherapy and radiotherapy treatments will temporarily or permanently stop periods, leading to menopause at a young age. Whether or not this happens will depend on how old you are, how close you are to natural menopause, the dose and type of chemotherapy, and the duration and location of radiotherapy. Most cancer care professionals are very knowledgeable about the potential effects of treatments they give, and this will be discussed at the time, so you should get some warning that the treatment may lead to early menopause. In some young women, the ovaries do start to work again after cancer treatments, even if there is a delay in the return of periods, but they may not continue until the normal age and, even some years after the cancer treatments, early ovarian failure may occur. Menopause after cancer is further discussed in Chapter 6.

A type of menopause can be induced with medications too, in the hope that in reducing hormonal activity a medical complaint will improve. Injections or medicines taken regularly induce a 'pseudo-menopause', which ends once treatment ends. During the treatment period, women experience similar symptoms to those of a natural menopause and may be offered 'add-back' HRT to help these symptoms. This will usually be done under the guidance of a specialist.

Such conditions include:

◆ **Endometriosis** – suppressing the hormonal fluctuations of a regular cycle will inhibit the growth of endometriosis and hopefully reduce the chronic pain associated with it.

◆ **Premenstrual disorder** – severe premenstrual syndrome (PMS). You may be severely affected at certain times of the month and be offered treatment to suppress cycles in order to prevent PMS. This could be a long-term treatment or short term before considering surgery as a permanent solution.

◆ **Troublesome fibroids** – fibroids are benign growths that can lead to very heavy and painful periods. Before offering surgery, the gynaecologist may suggest hormonal suppression to shrink the fibroids, making surgery easier.

Consequences of an early menopause

Symptoms

Surgical menopause sometimes results in more intense menopausal symptoms than a natural menopause. The decline in oestradiol (oestrogen) levels is rapid following surgery and flushes and sweats commonly occur quite soon after surgery. Some women will not get any, others only mildly, but many describe them as frequent and intense. If the surgery is planned, it may be that hormone replacement therapy (HRT), if not contraindicated, is started very soon after surgery and so symptoms are prevented from developing, perhaps the optimum situation for women when this is possible.

If you have such surgery planned it is worth asking to be seen by a healthcare professional, who can advise about considering HRT. UK guidance from NICE (National Institute for Health and Care Excellence) agrees that women who are planning surgery that will induce menopause should be offered the opportunity for such a discussion before the operation. This may be with a well-informed general practitioner, a gynaecologist, or through referral to a specialist menopause service.

Young women may experience the same menopausal symptoms as older women, which are described in Chapter 1, but the impact on their lives may differ. Women going through menopause in their fifties have the double impact of ageing to consider, and this too affects expectations and how they feel. Young women almost have the reverse: they feel – and are – young in age, yet menopause is perceived to be a condition of midlife. They do not yet need to adapt to the ageing process and don't expect to. Young women sometimes describe being more impacted by the following symptoms:

◆ Vaginal dryness
◆ Dyspareunia – painful sex
◆ Sleep disturbance
◆ Low sex drive
◆ Flushes and sweats.

Other symptoms which young women may experience include:

◆ Tiredness
◆ Mood changes
◆ Irritability
◆ Skin and hair changes, dryness, itching
◆ Bladder symptoms, e.g. frequency, urgency.

Unlike surgical menopause, spontaneous premature ovarian insufficiency creeps up slowly on women, with gradual changes in periods and a slow onset of symptoms, if any. Often it is not the symptoms that make people seek help but concern about the lack of periods and the possibility of conceiving. The oral contraceptive pill masks natural periods and sometimes it is only when a woman comes off the pill to get pregnant that she realises there may be a problem. The contraceptive pill has not caused the problem, merely masked an underlying issue.

While many of these symptoms are classically related to hormone loss, many may also be attributable to life stresses or other medical conditions, so diagnosis and investigation is often delayed while other factors are taken into consideration. Ovarian insufficiency may be the last factor to be tested for and for many women it is a relief when finally hormonal tests indicate a cause for their symptoms, even if the diagnosis itself is not a welcome one. If you suspect hormonal symptoms and have episodes without periods, testing will probably be done earlier and be quite reliable. If you still see sporadic periods, hormonal tests may be misleading and lead to delayed diagnosis.

Diagnosis

Every time I saw my doctor, he did yet another test, to rule out illness. He never thought to check my hormones, he said I was too young for menopause.

Women report having to seek help on several occasions before being seriously investigated for POI. This is reasonable on the one hand because POI is not the most obvious cause of most symptoms in young women, but it leads to delay in diagnosis and treatment, including fertility support. If a woman sees a significant change in menstrual regularity and especially if she has no periods for more than three or four months, with no explanation, then POI should be considered. Blood tests are easy to do and, while not always conclusive, can offer an insight into ovarian activity and are the first step in identifying the problem. Further blood tests may be needed, but basic hormone levels of follicle stimulating hormone (FSH) are a starting point.

FSH levels fluctuate naturally during the menstrual cycle and gradually rise as ovarian activity ceases. After menopause FSH is raised, at whatever age you are. In young women, an elevated FSH is an indication of ovarian insufficiency and two or three successively high levels over two to three months is needed to make a diagnosis, along with menstrual changes, often no periods at all or very scanty ones. There is no agreed level of FSH which confirms POI, but most health professionals agree that at least two levels over 40 iu/l, around four to six weeks apart, confirms the diagnosis. This means that in the early stages, a woman may have several tests before this pattern appears. Fluctuating FSH levels, including some raised, indicates early stage POI. The test should be done on day two to five of the cycle if you still have periods (day one is the first day of your period).

Oestradiol (oestrogen) levels will fall as FSH rises, but again they fluctuate widely so are not usually used alone as a diagnostic tool. Once POI is suspected, a full hormonal assay including FSH, oestradiol and luteinising hormone may be performed to assess full hormonal function. This may be done at a later stage to the initial testing of the FSH levels as part of a more comprehensive assessment. At that stage, you may also be offered pelvic ultrasound (scan) to look directly at the ovaries by ultrasound, in particular to see if there is any follicular activity (production of eggs) as well as more tailored blood tests to check for anti-mullerian hormone (AMH) and autoantibodies. Autoantibodies may offer an explanation as to why the POI occurred and AMH may help with predicting the possibility of success using IVF (in vitro fertilisation).

Anti-mullerian hormone (AMH) is sometimes referred to as a test for ovarian reserve. AMH is produced by small ovarian follicles so measuring it is thought to reflect the size of the remaining egg supply. It is not recommended as a routine test for diagnosis of ovarian insufficiency as the results can be contradictory and not always useful. If you are seeking fertility support, it can be a useful test, as higher levels of AMH predict better response with IVF (in vitro fertilisation). However, low levels in young women (under 35 years) do not always predict poor response to IVF. AMH cannot give any information about the quality of eggs either. So the test is usually combined with others for fertility assessment and is usually done by a fertility specialist.

> ### Recommendation
>
> If it is suspected that you have menopause under the age of 40, make sure that you are offered at least two blood tests, possibly more, to confirm the diagnosis.

It is reasonable to have simple FSH tests initially then more comprehensive testing later, including genetic testing if you are under 30. At present there is no intervention that can be offered to change genetic susceptibility to POI, so the point of genetic testing is for information and to help with decision making, rather than offering any treatment to prevent it.

Understandably it is the short-term effects of ovarian insufficiency that worry women the most – lack of periods, symptoms, and effects on fertility. These issues are paramount as women are helped to understand the condition and find out what treatments are available. Psychological support is crucial and some women will need the support of a counsellor or peer support in order to process what can be a difficult diagnosis. This is discussed later in this chapter.

Long-term health

I did not realise that this [POI] could have a long-lasting effect on my health. I thought it was just all about periods and having a baby.

While women are settling into the management of their short-term symptoms and being supported psychologically if necessary, the healthcare professional will want to address long-term health needs following ovarian insufficiency and especially following surgical menopause. In particular you will need advice about preserving bone health (prevention of osteoporosis) and promoting good cardiovascular health (prevention of coronary heart disease) as both of these are known to be influenced by hormonal loss at a young age.

The younger you are, the more the need to plan for long-term good health. Much of the advice will be the same for all men and women, such as:

- Not smoking
- Maintaining a healthy weight
- Balanced diet, low in saturated fats and salt, rich in fruit and vegetables
- Regular exercise
- Keeping alcohol to reasonable limits.

Other advice will be more specific to women going through menopause, at whatever age, and is discussed in Chapter 2.

Osteoporosis

I take HRT, not just to help my symptoms but because I know it will protect my bones against osteoporosis. I have no intention of being at risk of hip fracture later in life – for me that's important.

All the advice given to women going through the menopause at the so-called 'usual' time of around 50 years is also relevant to young women, as are the risk factors which may contribute to bone loss (see Chapter 2). However, it is acknowledged that early ovarian loss itself has an adverse effect on bone density and increases the risk of osteoporosis later in life. Chapter 1 describes how menopause influences bone health and these effects are heightened in young women as the bone loss occurs earlier and the consequence of fracture may therefore be earlier too.

Women will have different underlying risks for osteoporosis, regardless of hormonal function, and early ovarian failure (or insufficiency) is a modifiable risk factor, in that replacement hormones may be given through HRT, if there are no contraindications to its use. This is why if you are undergoing planned surgical removal of ovaries you should discuss the use of HRT prior to the procedure. If you are advised not to use HRT for medical reasons, other bone health strategies should be considered along with a baseline bone densitometry (DEXA or bone scan) to assess risk. NICE Guidance reassures women that, while they are using HRT, bone density is preserved. For bone protection, HRT use should be considered long term, and if you are young, this usually means using it until around 50, the usual age of menopause, unless there are medical reasons to avoid it. This is supported by all medical authorities and is the recommendation from NICE Guidance.

Heart disease

Until this happened, I had no idea that hormones play a role in preventing heart disease in women – what an eye-opener!

Early studies of women undergoing surgical menopause demonstrated that losing ovarian function greatly increased the risk of heart disease later in life, in all women but especially in smokers. Natural menopause at a young age is also thought to increase cardiovascular risk and, in young women, replacing oestrogen as part of HRT soon after early menopause is considered to be cardioprotective, i.e. good for the heart. One of the reasons that women under 40 are advised to consider HRT until natural age of menopause is to minimise cardiovascular risk. You still need to include other healthy lifestyle measures, such as not smoking, limiting alcohol intake, regular exercise and maintaining a healthy weight, and as always the risks of using HRT must be balanced against the benefits for each individual. HRT benefits are discussed in Chapter 4. General lifestyle advice around menopause is relevant at all ages and can be found in Chapter 2.

Sexual and bladder health

I don't know who was more embarrassed, me or my GP – surely it should not be like that? It's normal isn't it?

Both the vagina and the bladder rely on oestrogen to maintain healthy function. Surgical menopause, in particular, can result in bladder and sexual symptoms if HRT is not offered. Typical symptoms may include:

- Frequency in needing to pass urine
- Needing to wee at night
- Vaginal discomfort – dryness and itching
- Pain on intercourse
- Decreased libido (sex drive).

Some women will not notice any of these, others may get some, and for a few women they may become a significant problem if not treated. Ideally, if you get these symptoms, you should be offered treatment before symptoms get too troublesome, either as HRT or, if that is not possible, local vaginal treatments. However, it is never too late to treat and women are encouraged to be bold and broach the topic with their healthcare professional (HCP). Unfortunately, not all HCPs are comfortable talking about intimate issues, although they most certainly should be – it is part of normal life! As a result they may not ask the direct questions to allow you to be open about the problem. Instead, you may need to raise it yourself, by asking questions such as these:

- Sex has become uncomfortable, can you suggest anything to help?
- I find myself going to the toilet much more often: is this normal? Can you help?
- My partner and I find sex hurts now. What can I do?
- My vagina is very sore: I need some help, please.
- My sex drive has lessened, and that troubles me. What can I do?

I was embarrassed [to discuss sex], *but I did not need to be. The doctor put me at ease.*

Studies repeatedly show that women put up with such symptoms for quite a while before seeking help and that clinicians may be bad at approaching this topic. Sexual function should be as easy to talk about with your HCP as any other problem you may have. HCPs are being encouraged to ask directly, but women report that lack of time in consultations, professionals who are young and male (and therefore difficult to discuss this with), and the attitude that sex is an 'added bonus' rather than a relationship need, all contribute to obstacles in discussions.

Sex drive (libido) in women is influenced by far more than just hormones and although the lack of oestrogen undoubtedly contributes to poor sex drive, there is a lot more to improving it than simply prescribing HRT. Vaginal dryness itself can lead to a lack of arousal and a subsequent enjoyment of sex, meaning that next time your desire is lower, you are not so aroused, it is painful … and so the cycle continues. Breaking the cycle of vaginal dryness sometimes helps sex drive, so the first step is to ensure that the vagina is comfortable. Women who are not offered HRT or local vaginal oestrogen after surgical menopause at a young age often say that vaginal dryness was the start of their loss of interest in sex.

If you are taking HRT in the form of patches, gels and tablets for your early menopause, it will help vaginal symptoms, but vaginal dryness is easy to treat, and there is a choice of types of vaginal oestrogen you can use. These are discussed in Chapter 4. Even if you cannot use conventional HRT, you may be able to use vaginal oestrogen and if you really can't there are non-hormonal moisturisers and lubricants to help. Non-hormonal choices are discussed in Chapter 3.

Testosterone

Testosterone is a female hormone, although we often perceive it as being exclusively a male one. Ovaries release both oestrogen and testosterone. Women continue to make testosterone right up to menopause, although over the years levels will decline with age. When this happens, many women adapt and hardly notice the effect on sex drive. However, in young women who undergo surgical menopause, when the ovaries are removed the body loses its testosterone production rapidly and, with conventional HRT, it is not replaced.

If you experience natural menopause, even early, you may not always notice the effects of declining testosterone.

Actual testosterone levels may not correlate with sexual desire, but rapidly falling levels sometimes lead to problems with sex drive and also energy and general drive. As not all women seem to be sensitive to this fall, testosterone is not routinely used after surgical menopause, and many women do not need it. Some, however, would benefit from testosterone as well as oestrogen therapy so if for an individual this is an issue, it is worth asking your health professional to consider prescribing additional testosterone.

In the UK, however, there is a problem with this: there is no easily available product containing testosterone that is licensed for women. There are products licensed for men but the doses are too high for women if they are used in the same way. Studies have shown that if women use the same medicines, but at a much lower dose, it can be effective. So specialists will sometimes prescribe the male gels to women, on the understanding that they use the daily dose for a man over a period of at least a week. This is described as using a medicine 'off license', and not all HCPs are happy to do it, although it is worth noting that in 2015, NICE, in its helpful guidance on menopause management, suggested that off-license use of testosterone could be considered. If your own HCP does not wish to prescribe it or feels a lack of confidence in doing so, it is worth asking to see a specialist who is familiar with its use. Those working in this field hope that, in time, manufacturers will see the need to develop a product specifically for women.

As with all women, of all ages, desire for sex hinges not just on hormones but is influenced by relationships, health, stress, tiredness, environment (holidays often help!) and, of course, good communication. Hormones play a role and if the sex issue remains a problem, despite good hormones, you may wish to seek help from a sex therapist or psychosexual doctor or counsellor. Such experts can be found through your GP or by searching for 'psychosexual therapist' online, in your area. Be sure to use a fully qualified therapist. Look for one who is a member of the College of Sexual and Relationship Therapists (COSRT) or the Institute of Psychosexual Medicine (IPM). See the Resources section.

Treatment

I was not rushed into treatment; I had time to consider which I might prefer and to come to terms with even needing long-term hormone replacement.

Once a diagnosis is confirmed, and women understand

the implications to health and fertility, they will be offered hormone replacement. For most women, this will be in the form of hormone replacement therapy (HRT) and the types offered will be similar to those given to women experiencing menopause at the average age of 50. As with all women, the type and route of HRT should be discussed and your preference about patches, tablets or gels, all of which are suitable for young women, should be taken into account. Occasionally there will be medical reasons why one route or type is more appropriate than another, and this is discussed in Chapter 4, along with descriptions of the different ways in which the treatment can be used.

When the doctor said that I might be on HRT for twenty years, I hesitated, then she reminded me that if my ovaries were working properly I would have natural hormones until then anyway, so that reassured me.

Providing there are no medical reasons not to, HRT will be suggested until the normal age of menopause, so a young woman may well be on HRT for many years. It is important to understand that a young woman almost always needs oestrogen replacement and that the risks of not using it (e.g. cardiovascular disease, osteoporosis) usually means that the benefits generally outweigh small risks or side effects. Women should have the opportunity to discuss the benefits and risk of treatment on an individual basis. The situation may be different for a woman who has become menopausal as a result of cancer treatment, and this is discussed in Chapter 6. Risks and benefits of HRT are discussed in

Chapter 4, including the different risks and benefits for young women.

I am nineteen years old; I really don't want to be on HRT. What will my friends think?

NICE Guidance for health professionals has looked at whether it is reasonable to use the oral contraceptive (the pill) instead of HRT, but there has not been a great deal of research in this area. NICE say that young women may choose the pill instead, assuming that they don't want to be pregnant and they have no other medical reasons to avoid it. HRT may be better for blood pressure, but in young, healthy, non-smoking women, this is unlikely to be a significant issue; and it will certainly help prevent the bone loss associated with premature ovarian insufficiency. In practical terms, young women often choose the pill over HRT in order to be similar to their peers and to keep life simple. In the UK, there is the added advantage that contraception is free, whereas you pay a prescription charge for HRT.

Fertility

If someone had told me this was going to happen, I would have had a baby much sooner; it is so unfair.

I came off the pill to have a baby and had no periods. Now I'm menopausal – all those years on the pill and now this.

I really want to support my wife, but having kids was part of my life plan. What happens now?

In our culture having children is really important, so I let my parents believe it was my 'fault' so that they do not look badly on my wife. (Male partner)

Losing the option to have a baby, or another baby, can be devastating. Even if the family is theoretically 'complete', having the choice taken away is difficult to cope with, for both men and women. With support and over time, you may come to terms with it, and options are available for women who want to try to have a child or an additional child. It is not an easy path and you will need a referral to a specialist fertility clinic. If you want treatment on the NHS, there are strict criteria, which vary according to where you live. Some areas will not offer NHS treatment if you already have one child or if your partner has a child in another relationship. This may seem very unfair, and you can ask to be treated as an 'exceptional case', but battling with the bureaucracy of the NHS is never easy, and can itself be an uphill struggle. There are also age restrictions in most areas, usually 40, but sometimes 35. If you can afford to be seen privately, your options will be much broader, with finance and time constraints being the only limiting factors.

Is there a chance of a 'miracle' baby?'

You may have heard of women getting pregnant despite being 'menopausal'. This is because ovaries do not always stop suddenly and even some years after apparently stopping to work, they may occasionally get a burst of normal activity. Some women will spontaneously ovulate on occasion and pregnancy can occur – although it is quite unusual. Studies suggest that up to 5 to 10 per cent of women with POI will eventually get pregnant – on their own, without treatment from a fertility doctor. Statistically, this means that it is unlikely but possible for a rare pregnancy to occur once the diagnosis of POI is made.

Once the follicles in the ovary fail to mature, as in true ovarian failure, there is currently no effective treatment that is likely to result in a pregnancy (with your own eggs). If you are in the early stages of POI, it may be possible to stimulate your own ovaries through IVF (in vitro fertilisation). You should seek the advice of a fertility specialist to assess the likelihood of success before committing to a costly IVF cycle.

Deciding to have egg donation was difficult, but my partner was supportive and now we have two lovely girls that I gave birth to in a normal way.

Egg donation is a highly successful treatment, which is where you receive the implantation of an embryo that has been created with your partner's sperm and a donor's egg (usually anonymous). If successful, you carry the baby to term and deliver it normally as a mother. From a legal perspective, you are the birth mother. Referral to a fertility service will be necessary so that appropriate assessments and investigations can be performed, along with the IVF procedures. Egg donation is not usually available on the NHS and there can be a wait for donated eggs, delaying treatment further.

Other options include surrogacy and adoption, both of which need careful consideration and expert advice. You will find information about where to find out more in the Resources section. If you want up-to-date and accurate information about fertility treatments, take a look at the website www.HFEA.gov.uk, which outlines all the options and includes advice on how to access them as well as important issues to consider when doing so.

If the surgical removal of ovaries is planned (e.g. for cancer), oocytes (eggs) can sometimes be retrieved prior to the treatment, if time allows. These can then be cryopreserved (frozen), stored and used later for in vitro fertilisation (IVF). This a complex issue with varying success rates. If you already have a partner, it may be suggested that you have IVF leading to frozen embryos, which are then stored until you are healthy enough to allow pregnancy, when the embryos are implanted into your womb. Ovarian tissue may be cryopreserved (frozen) too, but this is mainly at research stage rather than in practical clinical use – you may read about it in the press.

I did want children, but you adapt to what life throws at you. No children now but a wonderful, full life that I would have missed out on if I did have children.

Remaining childfree is in some women's life plan, but for others, it is an option they would not have considered. Society leads us to believe that having children is the norm and the decision not to have children may be regarded as odd. Yet many, many women choose not to have children and life is good – very good. Perhaps a bigger issue is the choice being taken away, a situation being imposed on you and the lack of control over it. Adjustment to the lack of choice is a painful process, and it can help to talk this through with a counsellor as feelings of anger, sadness and grief for what could have been are normal.

If you are particularly young, perhaps a teenager and not yet ready to even consider starting a family, you should remember that medical research is advancing all the time and that options may be open to you that at present we don't even know about. Freezing of parts of ovarian tissue before cancer treatment are in early stages of research and show promise, along with stem cell research which is at a very early stage.

Psychological issues

Menopause is often associated with ageing. I am not old, but being described as menopausal makes me feel old.

I am young, my mum is menopausal: how can I possibly be the same as my mum?

Every woman's experience of menopause is unique, at whatever age it occurs. If you are young, going through the process of diagnosis, accepting it, and planning for the future all take time. It is not surprising that you may need extra support psychologically. If you are not offered counselling or support, and feel it would be beneficial, do ask how you can access it. This may be through a specialist menopause service or a counsellor with a specific interest.

Women sometimes describe feelings about menopause that reflect society's misconceptions – to do with ageing, defining femininity or sexuality, or that menopause is a disease. Such attitudes are not helpful and for some women psychological help such as peer support or counselling may be useful. Others describe feeling isolated following diagnosis, since the condition is not visible and others around you may fail to understand the impact. You may need ongoing medical support, which can make you feel 'medicalised', even though medical treatments are designed to keep you healthy rather than to 'treat' the menopause itself. Post diagnosis, it is the consequences of menopause that you need help with, to ensure that your body benefits from the female hormones that you would be getting if your ovaries were working efficiently. Repeated medical consultations may make you feel different from apparently healthy peers. Much of what you hear can seem negative and can be emotionally difficult. Your partner or your family may not understand the implications fully and may also want extra information and support.

For some, the diagnosis is a relief, as you finally find out what is wrong and can take positive action to improve health. If supported, your immediate reaction of shock and, perhaps, distress, can turn into a plan of action and, eventually, acceptance. As this process can take time it is important that health professionals don't rush consultations and that they give you a chance to ask questions and make treatment decisions.

Summary

The medical, personal and social situations of women experiencing a young menopause, whether it is naturally occurring, due to surgery or as a result of disease, vary considerably from woman to woman. It is to be hoped that medical support is improving and that you will be able to seek a referral to a specialist if you feel that you are not getting the help, treatment and support that you need.

There is increasing recognition that you may need different kinds of help at various times, whether that is support for the diagnosis, fertility support, advice on long-term health needs or work/social needs, and you may have to ask for help when you need it. Excellent communication with medical practitioners is a two-way process, and it often helps to prepare issues you want to discuss.

During the diagnosis you might experience feelings of shock, numbness, then anger, low mood or feelings of despair. This is a normal reaction to a negative life event and, gradually, acceptance and adaptation will come. It really helps to have a supportive person alongside, whether that is a friend, partner or health professional.

There will be lots of questions you will want to ask and issues to consider. Here is a reminder:

- Why is it happening? It may not always be possible to say why.
- What is the short-term plan? How will I feel, what will happen to me?

◆ What is the long-term plan? How can I look after my health, particularly bone and heart health, but also sexual health and fertility?

◆ Can I use HRT and, if so, what types and for how long?

◆ Is there anything else I should be doing, e.g. bone scans, dietary advice?

◆ Where can I access support if I need it?

Frequently asked questions about young menopause/premature ovarian insufficiency

1 *I feel very isolated. I don't know anyone else with this – where can I get advice?*

When you are given this diagnosis at a young age it can make you feel very alone. Your clinician should offer time for discussion and questions, perhaps offering counselling too if needed. Most menopause advice is aimed at mid-age women and you may feel that this is just not appropriate for you. Take a look at www.daisy-network.org.uk – a website aimed specifically at young women.

2 *I am 36 years old. Do I need different tests for menopause than a woman who is 50?*

Yes, you will need a complete evaluation to assess hormone function and look for other reasons why your periods may have stopped. It may take a few months to reach a final diagnosis and then treatment will be discussed with you. You will need ongoing support in a different way to an older woman and may need psychological support alongside medical treatment while you understand the diagnosis and the impact it may have, for example, on fertility and future health.

3 *It looks like I could be on HRT for more than fifteen years: is this really OK?*

If your ovaries stop working properly and you are under 40 years old, you will be recommended HRT for many years, until at least the average of menopause, unless there are medical reasons not to use it. This is because the many years you could face without your own circulating oestrogen can have an adverse effect on your body, particularly the skeleton and cardiovascular system. By taking HRT, you are simply replacing the hormones your body can no longer make and this, alongside long-term healthy lifestyle measures, protects your future health. When you get to the average age of menopause, you can choose whether or not to stay on HRT, by assessing your health and balancing any potential risks.

4 *I have been told I have premature ovarian insufficiency. Is the same as early menopause?*

The terms 'premature ovarian insufficiency' (POI) and 'early menopause' describe very similar changes in your body. POI is a more accurate description when, in young women, the ovaries stop working effectively and periods lessen or stop. It can be hard to know the precise moment that 'menopause' (the last ever period) occurs, as hormonal function can fluctuate sometimes over many years, so the term POI is more appropriate. If you have had your ovaries removed by an operation, the term 'early menopause' is more accurate.

5 *I have planned surgery to remove my ovaries. Should I talk about whether I may need HRT now or wait until afterwards?*

If you are under 45 and have an operation planned to remove your ovaries, I think you should have the opportunity to discuss the possible impact of symptoms and possible use of HRT beforehand. The younger you are, the more important this discussion will be, particularly in relation to long-term health. You will need to know if there are any reasons you cannot use HRT and if so how you can access help for symptoms, if they should arise. You might want to ask who will offer HRT after the operation: will it be the surgeon or will you be discharged to the GP for after-care? Being prepared will help you feel equipped to face the surgery more positively, knowing you can access support afterwards if you need it.

6 *I want to talk about fertility and whether or not I can even get pregnant; and, if not, what are my options? How do I get to see someone who can discuss this with me?*

If you are under the care of a specialist when diagnosed with premature ovarian insufficiency, they should be able to have this discussion with you. Often working closely with fertility experts, they can refer you for a consultation to consider your options. They may not actually offer fertility treatments themselves but will know how to access them. Otherwise, you can ask your GP to refer you for an initial fertility consultation. In the private sector, you can often self-refer for an opinion and information consultation.

7 *My ovaries have stopped working at age 36 but I feel absolutely fine. I already have children so that's not a problem to me, so why should I take HRT? I just want to move on with life.*

At 36 years old, you are young, and if confirmed to have ovarian insufficiency, you will be recommended HRT until around the age of natural menopause. This is because for many young women the health risks of taking nothing are higher than the risks of taking HRT. You need to consider the benefits to your heart and bones in particular that you will miss out on if you do not use HRT. These are silent changes in your body, so you will not be aware of them. Finding the right HRT for you may take a few months, but the benefits once established will last much longer.

chapter 6

Menopause after cancer

Living with induced menopause

Having cancer was dreadful, then just as you think you are over the worst, you are knocked back by menopause ... I was just not prepared for that, on top of everything else.

The previous chapter discussed early menopause or premature ovarian insufficiency. I talked about surgical menopause and described it as 'induced', because the menopause is brought on by the intentional removal of ovaries through an operation, sometimes because of cancer. Induced menopause can also be caused medically by the use of cancer treatment that aims to improve the rate of survival but has the side effect of causing menopause, even in young women. In this chapter, we explore which treatments may commonly cause induced menopause, how it may affect you, and what you can do about it without adversely affecting your cancer risk.

Getting to the end of treatment is a milestone, it has felt so long.

It is good news that cancer survival rates are improving, and with modern therapies many women can expect to live far beyond the initial cancer treatment phase.

Like most women who have undergone cancer treatments, you look forward to them ending and moving on with life as normal. The disruption caused by undergoing surgery, radiotherapy and chemotherapy cannot be underestimated and most cancer units are excellent at supporting women through this difficult time. You will have completed an intense treatment programme where each phase is well researched, each course of therapy a stepwise approach towards recovery, and finally you have got there. The end of treatment is often a celebration, and you may be starting to make plans for a healthy future, including going back to work, back to social activities and planning holidays or other events. Over time, follow-up visits to cancer centres reduce and you may be discharged back to the care of your family doctor or with only annual visits to the cancer centre. You may not have any follow-up planned at all. Fewer hospital visits are seen as a progression towards normality – surely a positive step.

Yet it can be at this time, just when life begins to take shape again, that symptoms of menopause may occur. Perhaps you were warned that your treatment might lead to loss of periods, you may have had a discussion about early menopause and you may have been given a leaflet about managing menopausal symptoms, but until it happens to you, its effects are often underestimated. Of course cancer has taken priority, both in your mind and that of the doctors treating you, but now you want to live life, get back to normality, and perhaps you are not expecting menopause to be much of an impact compared to the cancer treatments. So when it happens, you may be surprised or even shocked at the impact menopausal symptoms can have, the way they make you feel physically and emotionally and their effect on everyday life. You may have anticipated a short transition time that you would be able to cope with, but the reality can be much harder. Add to that the fact that your cancer can make it more difficult to find suitable treatments and it is not surprising if you find yourself in the midst of troublesome symptoms, being offered little help. Sometimes the best-intentioned medical staff seem to have little to offer.

I knew menopause was a consequence of my treatment but until it happened, I had no idea what to expect. I probably didn't listen anyway, I was consumed with getting through the cancer, I was not thinking ahead at all.

Why does it happen?

In order to treat my cancer, the ovaries were removed surgically, so I knew I would be menopausal straight away. I had time to ask questions and prepare for the inevitable symptoms.

I had been warned that the chemotherapy might cause loss of ovarian function, but it did not happen immediately so I thought maybe I had got away with it. It was months afterwards that my periods finally stopped and symptoms started. Then it felt like they never stopped!

I was advised to take medication that put me into a type of false menopause, so although it meant the cancer treatment

could be more effective, it made me go through all the
symptoms of menopause and quite abruptly.

Surgery

If the ovaries are removed as part of cancer surgery, or
if healthy ovaries are removed in order to minimise the
risk of cancer, you will go into a sudden menopause.
The younger you are, the greater the impact this might
have, both on how you feel and on your future health. If
you were already close to menopause when the surgery
took place, you might not notice the effects so much,
as your body will already have started the changes associated with menopause. If you are younger, you will
notice the changes more acutely and might start to
get menopausal symptoms soon after your operation.
Flushes might be the first sign of symptoms, along with
night sweats, and then other symptoms like tiredness
and mood changes might become noticeable. Sex
might be affected both because of vaginal changes and
because of changes in desire or libido.

The types of surgery that will put you into sudden
menopause are:

◆ Hysterectomy with bilateral salpingo-oophorectomy
(womb, tubes and ovaries removed), whether this is
done through laparoscopy (telescope) or with a scar
on the bikini line.

◆ BSO, bilateral salpingo-oophorectomy, where both
tubes and ovaries are removed.

If one or both ovaries are left behind, your menopause

should not be so sudden, and may not, in fact, be any different to what you would have experienced had you not had surgery. Occasionally the menopause happens a bit earlier than it would have done otherwise and you will be advised to seek help if you start to experience symptoms. Remember that, without a womb, you will not have the marker of periods to give you a clue that menopause is approaching, so it might only be symptoms that alert you.

If you have had notice of the surgery, in other words, it is not an emergency but planned surgery, you should have the opportunity to discuss management of your menopause in advance. Questions to ask your gynaecologist include:

- Are both ovaries being removed?
- Will I need HRT and be able to use it?
- If I can't use HRT, what options do I have for symptoms?
- If I am to start HRT, who will prescribe it, hospital or GP?
- If I can take HRT, can we discuss types and routes so that I am ready?
- When should I start it?

Chemotherapy and radiotherapy

Fortunately, I was warned the treatment might cause menopause; it did not come as a shock.

Cancer treatments affect hormones in different ways,

so your experience may not be the same as someone else's, but there are patterns and known effects. For some, it will be the cancer treatment itself that leads to ovarian failure, or suppression. For example, particular chemotherapy, for example for breast cancer, is known to cause the ovaries to stop working and so lead to early menopause. Your periods may stop gradually during chemotherapy and then return once treatment is finished or the effect may be permanent, depending on the type and dose of chemotherapy you have had. Your periods may return months or years after chemotherapy has finished. Your cancer doctors will have discussed the likelihood of this happening, but cannot always predict exactly what will happen to an individual. Generally, the closer you are to the age of natural menopause when you start treatment the more likely it is that your periods will stop during chemotherapy and that the effect will be permanent. This means that once treatment is finished, you may have the onset of menopause, with all the accompanying symptoms. It may be difficult to know whether it is the chemotherapy directly causing your symptoms or the effect of menopause as there is much overlap in the type of symptoms you may experience. Menopausal symptoms may not start until after the chemotherapy has finished and can go on for quite a long time afterwards, even well after cancer treatment is over.

Radiotherapy to your pelvic area such as for gynaecological cancers, which includes cervical, ovarian and womb cancers, will also have an effect on ovarian function, often leading to menopause. Periods will gradually stop and menopausal symptoms might occur, either while treatment is underway or later on. Sometimes, especially if you are a young woman, you may have been offered an operation to try to move the ovaries out of the way of the radiation in order to reduce the risk, but this is not always successful and periods may still stop. It may take several months before you notice menopausal symptoms, but the change in periods is often the first sign. If you have loss of ovarian function (or menopause) due to radio-therapy, it is usually permanent and often accompa-nied by troublesome symptoms, similar to those of a normal menopause, but sometimes more severe. It is difficult to predict how you will experience menopause after radiotherapy and it is important to remember that some symptoms will be caused by the local effects of radiotherapy, particularly physical ones to the pelvic area and vagina, while more general symptoms like flushes and sweats will be menopausal.

Radiotherapy for gynaecological cancers can lead to changes in the vagina and bladder, and you may find that sex is uncomfortable. The tissues of the vagina may have become fragile and bleed easily and may also be sore or itchy. Vaginal discharge may change and you may be susceptible to infections, which can be bother-some and for which you will need treatment, usually in the form of vaginal treatments or antibiotics. The loss of hormones caused by menopause can lead to vaginal changes too, some of which can be treated with local vaginal oestrogen. Whether or not you can use local vaginal oestrogen will depend on the type of cancer you had and its staging (i.e. how advanced or how much it has spread). You will need to discuss this with your gynaecologist or cancer specialist. There are different types of vaginal oestrogens so it is important that you get the opportunity to discuss which might suit you. Local vaginal oestrogen is discussed more in Chapter 4. If you are unable to use local vaginal oestrogen, or if you want to try something without hormones first, there are several non-hormonal moisturisers and lubricants available, both to be purchased and prescribed. These are also discussed more in Chapter 4.

As a result of radiotherapy, the vagina can become narrower and shorter, so your cancer nurses will have advised about the use of dilators or vibrators to maintain vaginal flexibility. This may be uncomfortable but is paramount for maintaining sexual function, and the use of a good lubricant will help to make them more comfortable. You should always feel able to discuss this important topic with your healthcare professional as help is available and it is often a very challenging part of the recovery after radiotherapy for gynaecological cancers. It is not just the physical effects that are important: it is normal to experience emotional changes that will influence enjoyment of sex, and many of the cancer charities have help and information about this important topic. See the Resources chapter for more information.

Breast cancer treatments

To many, it seems logical that there will be an effect

on hormones if the cancer is gynaecological; after all, that's where the hormones are. If you have had breast cancer, you may not always understand the link, and yet it is very likely that you will go into menopause or experience menopause-like side effects from your treatment. Common chemotherapy regimens used to treat breast cancer often directly affect your ovaries, leading to your periods stopping and then to early menopause, especially if you are close to the age of natural menopause when diagnosed.

Chemotherapy brought its own side effects, then menopause hit – double symptoms just when you feel at your worst, at least with chemo you can see an end to it.

On top of this, you may have been given long-term medication to prevent a return of cancer, and these have a hormonal effect, often resulting in symptoms very similar to menopause. Often described as 'endocrine treatments' because they affect the hormone or endocrine system of the body, they are given to you if your breast cancer is oestrogen receptor positive. This means that cancer has receptors within the cell that bind to the hormone oestrogen and stimulate cancer to grow. Not all breast cancers are hormone receptor positive, so not all women need this endocrine type of long-term treatment.

The endocrine treatments block the hormonal effects and, as a result, the breast cancer is thought less likely to return or grow. If you are not menopausal at the time of diagnosis and the treatment does not lead to menopause, the breast specialists may choose to temporarily cause a type of menopause using medication in order to reduce the amount of oestrogen circulating in your body and allow the use of particular cancer treatments. This is usually a monthly injection that will suppress your ovaries and you will feel as if you are menopausal. It is often described as 'pseudo-menopause'. Once the injections are stopped, periods will often return, unless you were close to age 50 when they started, in which case you will probably transition into natural menopause and not notice a precise time when you became naturally menopausal. While using the injections, you will experience the common changes that menopause brings, including symptoms. In some cases you may be offered surgical removal of ovaries instead of monthly injections, which would lead to permanent menopause and needs careful consideration because it cannot be reversed. If you are close to natural age of menopause, you and your cancer doctor may conclude that this is a reasonable choice.

Endocrine treatments include:

- Tamoxifen
- Aromatase inhibitors, such as anastrozole, exemestane and letrozole
- LH (luteinising hormone) blockers.

All of these treatments can lead to menopause-like symptoms as well as the onset of the menopause itself, which is often caused by the chemotherapy. This is why the treatment of breast cancer may result in you seeking help for menopausal symptoms. Many symptoms will be the same as those of a typical menopause, but treatment may be more difficult because it is unlikely that you will be able to use hormone replacement therapy (see Chapter 4).

Symptoms

I have no idea what is caused by the side effects of tamoxifen and what by my menopause, but it is all awful.

I know many women don't want HRT but, believe me, not being able even to consider it is far worse.

Many of the symptoms associated with menopause after cancer will be the same as for normal menopause, but the impact may be different. Some symptoms may be more severe: for example, flushes and sweats are worsened by tamoxifen; joint aches can be a side effect of aromatase inhibitors or a menopausal symptom; and either treatment can worsen vaginal dryness and be a result of ageing or of menopause. You may find it hard to know if what you are experiencing are menopausal symptoms or are side effects of the treatment, but you will certainly know the effect they are having and may perhaps seek help. Those clinicians trying to help you will look at your symptoms and offer treatment where possible, whatever the underlying cause. Unlike in the case of natural menopause, they will often not be able to treat the underlying lack of oestrogen with HRT, because the cancer specialists specifically want oestrogen avoided in order to enhance the cancer care and reduce future risk.

It is useful to note that some gynaecological cancers are not specifically hormone-related, so if that is the case with your type of cancer, you might be able to use HRT following treatment. After many gynae cancers you may be able to use HRT to relieve menopausal symptoms or use local vaginal oestrogen to improve vaginal dryness and relieve painful sex. Speak to your gynae-oncologist.

Troublesome symptoms and treatment options

Flushes and sweats so intense that I have to leave the room: what on earth can I do?

My vaginal dryness doesn't just affect sex, it's sore all the time.

If only I could sleep – my sweats keep me awake all night.

Any menopausal symptom, as discussed in the chapter about normal menopause (Chapter 1), may arise when menopause results from cancer treatments. In particular, it is often the following that are the most troublesome:

◆ Flushes and sweats, day and night
◆ Tiredness
◆ Vaginal soreness and itching
◆ Painful sex.

When you discuss your symptoms, you will be offered some of the treatments given to women who have not had cancer, but probably not HRT, except possibly vaginal oestrogen, which you may be able to use under the supervision of your specialist. Non-hormonal treatments will be offered, some of which are only available through a specialist clinic, others from your GP. For more detailed information about each of these, see Chapter 3. Here is a summary of the options:

1 SSRIs and SNRIs

Selective serotonin reuptake inhibitors (SSRIs) and serotonin-norepinephrine reuptake inhibitors (SNRIs) are types of antidepressant that have been found to have the added effect of improving flushes and sweats. Examples of SSRIs are fluoxetine, citalopram and paroxetine; an example of SNRI is venlafaxine.

Note: You should not take paroxetine or fluoxetine if you are also taking tamoxifen, as these medicines can interfere with each other and potentially cause the tamoxifen to be less effective.

2 Clonidine

This tablet is used for high blood pressure and migraine and is also licensed for use to relieve hot flushes.

3 Gabapentin

Gabapentin is a medication used to treat neurological disorders such as seizures and neuropathic pain. In specialist clinics, it may be suggested for relief of severe flushes.

Over-the-counter products

In Chapter 3, I discussed non-hormonal products that

are available to buy, and looked at the evidence for their effectiveness. You may be thinking of using some of these for your symptoms of induced menopause. A potential problem with these is that there is little scientific research to show that they are safe to use after cancer. That does not mean they are necessarily unsafe, simply that we do not have the assurance that they will not interact with cancer treatments or stimulate the growth of previously treated cancer. Of the popular ones you can buy, most specialists will suggest avoiding the following after cancer because of unknown effects:

- Black cohosh
- Sage
- Isoflavones e.g. red clover / soya
- St John's wort.

Cognitive Behavioural Therapy

Cognitive behavioural therapy (CBT) is also discussed in depth in Chapter 3 and much of the research has been done looking at groups of women experiencing flushes and sweats after breast cancer, so it is very pertinent here too. CBT helps you to focus on your thoughts, feelings and behaviours in relation to your symptoms and helps you to adapt or cope with them. CBT is sometimes available through the NHS, is available privately, and can also be used as a type of 'self-help' strategy using handbooks and workbooks – see Resource section for examples and Chapter 3 for a more detailed outline of CBT.

Vaginal treatments

Vaginal symptoms were rarely discussed with me, yet they caused me such anxiety. Once I was given advice about treatment, I could finally do something about it.

I did not realise that vaginal oestrogen treatments were different to HRT. If only that was explained to me earlier.

Specific vaginal treatments are discussed in chapters 3 and 4. In relation to menopause after cancer, the primary issue is whether it is safe to use local vaginal oestrogen or whether it may affect future cancer risk. Vaginal oestrogen is very weakly absorbed and only influences the vaginal area of the body. If you have vaginal dryness, causing painful lovemaking, itching or burning, discuss vaginal treatments with your clinician. The final decision will usually lie with your oncologist (cancer doctor) but a gynaecologist may assess whether you would benefit from this treatment and your GP can certainly start the discussion. After gynaecological cancers such as cervical, ovarian and early stage endometrial (womb), low-dose vaginal oestrogen may be recommended if non-hormonal vaginal treatments are not sufficient to improve symptoms. The situation is more complex with breast cancer and there is divided opinion even among health professionals. The decision to use vaginal oestrogen after breast cancer will depend on the medication you are using long term to prevent recurrence, the type of cancer you had, as well as how long ago the cancer was treated and if there has been a recurrence. You should be able to have this discussion with your oncologist, which can help you to make the right choices.

Getting help

They [menopausal symptoms] *did not seem something to trouble the cancer clinic with, yet my GP, though sympathetic and understanding, was not very knowledgeable and there did not seem to be anywhere else to turn.*

As soon as you say you have had cancer, you know your treatment choices are limited, but sometimes you just want to at least discuss the options.

You may find it difficult to get the help you need for these symptoms because you may not be regularly attending the cancer clinic and your general practitioner may not have the specialist knowledge required to advise on treatments, that is with a good understanding of their effects on future cancer risk. In any case, it is also true that medical treatments are limited because there has not been a great deal of research in this area. That does not mean that there is no help available, however. Sometimes the support of a knowledgeable healthcare professional can be both reassuring and therapeutic even when no medical treatment is offered. You can ask to be referred back to your cancer specialist to discuss management of menopause and vaginal dryness and, in some areas, there will be specific menopause clinics who will liaise with cancer specialists to ensure consistency of care for both conditions.

You will, of course, want to be sure that any treatments offered for menopause are not to the detriment of your cancer treatment, so taking the time to find the right specialist is time well spent. In Chapter 8, there is information about how to find a specialist and your GP may also be able to recommend someone.

Women I have seen tell me that menopausal symptoms are often worse than they anticipated and that help was difficult to source. If you have had cancer, then you of all people are not going to risk harming treatment response by trying medicines that might interact or do harm. Occasionally, you may feel that the side effects of the long-term cancer treatments are so bad that you think about taking something to alleviate them. Before doing this, however bad a particular treatment make you feel, ask your oncologist (cancer doctor) to give you an honest review of its benefits – only then can you decide if the potential benefits are enough to keep you on it. Occasionally the oncologist will suggest an alternative cancer prevention treatment, in the hope of finding one that might suit you better or has fewer side effects, but with little loss of cancer prevention. If you have been discharged from your cancer centre it would be reasonable to ask to be referred back for this type of discussion, however long ago your treatment stopped. Most clinics know that you do not want unnecessary repeat appointments just in order to be told that all is well, so they have a system of open referral if problems arise. This is not just if you think the cancer has returned: an appointment can often be made to discuss ongoing effects of the cancer treatments as you live your life and this may include the effects on menopausal symptoms.

In the Resources section, you will find more places where you can seek help in relation to specific cancers and how to find support and information.

Frequently asked questions about menopause following cancer treatments

1 *My periods stopped during chemotherapy. Is that it now, will they never return?*

This is very individual. It will depend on how old you are when you have treatment and on the type and doses of chemotherapy you needed. If you are close to menopause age when you have treatment, it seems more likely that your periods will stop completely with chemotherapy. Sometimes the chemotherapy causes temporary damage to your ovaries, and periods may return, often six to twelve months after treatment has finished, sometimes much later than this.

2 *If I know they are going to be damaged can I freeze my ovaries before cancer treatment, to use at a later date?*

This is an area of promising research but it is not yet widely available in the UK. A small part of the ovarian tissue is removed and preserved. Later on, it can be transplanted back and if it starts working, may produce eggs. With IVF (in vitro fertilisation) techniques these may result in pregnancy. At present you are more likely to be offered a discussion round IVF and embryo preservation (if you have a partner) or possibly egg preservation (freezing), although again, egg freezing is still at early stages of research. Remember that all these discussions and any action to preserve fertility may take several weeks and that your specialist may recommend that cancer treatments start before then – you will need to openly discuss your options early on.

3 *I am grateful to my cancer specialist and the team, but feel a bit isolated with my symptoms now I am discharged. Yet I have ongoing menopausal symptoms. What can I do?*

This is a common feeling: you are moving on after the cancer but have to live with any ongoing menopausal symptoms. Please do ask for help, whether it is from your GP, the cancer nurse who was supporting you, or through various organisations (see the Resources section). Many of the symptoms you are experiencing can be addressed with the right support so please, don't just put up with them. Don't judge them as 'less important than the cancer', they are just different and still worth addressing if they can be. See Chapter 8 for advice on seeking support.

4 *I see lots of supplements advertised and I am very tempted to try them. Is it OK to do that?*

Many supplements are fine to use after cancer as they contain mainly vitamins or dietary supplements. Others, though, have herbal or even medical components and the safety of these for those who have had cancer may be less clear. Some supplements are known to have a potential interaction with long-term cancer prevention medicines like tamoxifen and should be avoided for this reason. Rather then just picking something off the shelf, perhaps speak to a pharmacist, your GP or your cancer nurse before buying supplements.

5 *How soon do menopause symptoms start if I have my ovaries removed by an operation?*

Every woman is different. If you were close to the age of natural menopause, e.g. 45 or older, you may not see a sudden onset of symptoms at all. You may experience a more gradual onset, as your hormones will already have been changing slowly even if you were still having periods. If you are younger, you may see symptoms like flushes and sweats quite quickly, perhaps within a couple of weeks and sometimes quite intensely. For some, they will happen only at night, for others, during the day as well. Other symptoms may be slower to develop, if they do at all. Even after surgical menopause, women vary individually and not all women will get the classic intense symptoms that you read about.

chapter 7

Menopause and work

The everyday challenge

It's embarrassing and difficult; I just want to hide my symptoms away.

My work area is covered in sticky notes to be sure I don't forget anything.

I am sure my boss does not understand – why would he?

I don't need 'special treatment', I just need to be allowed to get on and cope in the way I need, if that means a fan on the desk – is that so difficult?

Roughly half of all UK workers are women: in 2016, surveys reported that 70 per cent of women were working. The changes that you experience during the menopause transition inevitably have an effect not just on your personal life but also on how you feel and sometimes how you perform at work. As retirement ages slowly rise, women will have to work for many years beyond menopause before they reach pension age. Managers rarely discuss menopause and you may feel that, as a personal matter, it is not their business anyway. Sometimes, simple, small adjustments by an employer and an acknowledgement that menopause exists can make working through it much easier. You should not have to hide your symptoms and employers need to be aware that conditions at work may either exacerbate or alleviate the problem. An honest, private discussion between you and your manager may make work life much more manageable and avoid the misunderstandings that could otherwise arise.

> Surveys show that the majority of women are unwilling to disclose menopause-related health issues to line managers, most of whom are men or younger than them.
>
> Faculty of Occupational Medicine, 2016

> Women were less willing to disclose to managers who are male, or younger than them.
>
> Police Report, 2010

> Poor ventilation, high working temperatures (hot work), unsuitable clothing or uniforms, and some protective equipment can aggravate common menopausal symptoms such as hot flushes and sweating, affecting workers' comfort and health.
>
> Trades Union Congress, 2003

Increasingly, menopause is being recognised as an important work issue and various organisations have issued guidance to their members, e.g. Trades Union Congress (TUC) and UNISON, as well as numerous professional bodies such as the police, teaching unions and health unions. The Faculty of Occupational Medicine, a medical body with a remit to examine how health affects work, has issued guidance on this topic for all employers and workplaces (see the Resources section).

Corporations and organisations are beginning to recognise that well-being of staff and health at work issues must include menopause. It has become an issue for equality and diversity departments too, as gender-specific health concerns like menopause may inadvertently be treated differently to other health matters that affect both men and women.

For some, uniform might be a problem – the fabric, cut or weight might make symptoms worse and recurrent sweats might mean that you need frequent changes, and this becomes a problem if there is a limited supply of uniforms. Some organisations may allow you to wear something more comfortable, while others may have a procedure that takes several months. You might imagine that just asking for this to be taken into account would be enough to allow changes to happen, but for some people the bureaucracy inherent in an organisation means that it is not always easy.

Examples of uniform adjustments might include:

◆ Switching to cotton shirts from polo shirts or sweatshirts
◆ Having a uniform that can be layered and still looks professional
◆ Having more spare uniforms than is standard
◆ Being allowed to remove scarves or ties
◆ Provision of changing facilities.

Symptoms

> Women should feel as comfortable discussing
> menopausal symptoms as they would any other
> issues in the workplace.
>
> Dame Sally Davies, Chief Medical Officer, from *The Annual
> Report of the Chief Medical Officer 2014* (published 2015)

Coping with symptoms such as hot flushes, mood
changes and tiredness is hard at any time, but when they
happen at work it can cause you even more difficulty.
With friends and family, you may be happy to have the
odd joke about hormones and 'senior moments', but at
work you want to keep your professional demeanour
and maintain a confident and efficient approach. This
is understandable, and you may not need to mention it
at all. With small alterations to your work environment
and with minor adjustments within your day, you may
be able to continue with your job as normal. This will
depend on the control you have of your work environment, the severity of your symptoms and the actual job
you do. The seniority of your role may mean that you
can make subtle changes to your work pattern without
consulting others. Maybe you come in a little later and
work later, maybe you move your desk to a more airy
position. You can schedule meetings to suit you and be
in control of where and when they are held. You can
get to meetings early to avoid that rushed arrival and
prepare the room temperature to suit you.

In some jobs, you may be more restricted, even on
when you can leave your desk or have breaks. If you

are a teacher, you cannot always leave the classroom if a sweat breaks out; on the cash desk, breaks might be strictly scheduled; and in a busy office, you may have little or no control over the temperature of the room or whether or not you can open windows.

Involving a manager and making an official request is not easy, but look at it from their point of view; if you don't even make known the problems you are having, how can they help? Even if the question has not been asked before, your manager or employer has a duty to try to ensure that your workplace is suitable for you to work in. That means looking at a problem not previously addressed and working to find a solution.

Flushes

I spend my day arguing with young men that I need the air con up even though they are cold!

Having to leave my desk so that I can remove layers during a flush, that is annoying.

Flushes and sweats are the most common menopausal symptoms and ones that are often bothersome at work. At home, you have control over room temperature, the clothes you wear and taking breaks; at work, these may not be negotiable. You may be feeling embarrassed about it, not wanting to highlight the problem or draw attention to yourself. Your uniform or dress policy might mean wearing clothes that increase the chances of sweating, and during the actual flush, you may need to take a short break. People around may not even notice that you are uncomfortable; flushes are not always visible and even if they do see your redness or perspiration, they are probably too busy getting on with their own work to be fussed about it. Equally, if they see you apparently managing, they are unlikely to offer help or adjustments.

Tips for managing flushes at work:

◆ Request a desk fan to control your personal desk environment.

◆ Help colleagues to understand why you want the air conditioning turned up higher than they would like (it is often easier for them to add a layer than for you to cool down!).

◆ Consider your work wear and, if possible, allowing for 'unlayering' during a flush.

◆ Drink plenty of water to counteract the sweats and to help avoid headaches.

◆ Use a cooling mist in the heat of the flush – this will not stop the flush but may make you feel more comfortable.

◆ Allow more time to arrive at meetings: feeling rushed will worsen flushes.

◆ Try to avoid stress and anxiety at work – each may worsen flushes. Look at strategies to reduce these if this is a problem.

Tiredness, concentration and poor memory

Women report that, along with flushes and sweats, tiredness and lack of concentration and poor memory are some of the most troublesome menopausal symptoms at work. Night-time sweats, which often start before periods even change, can lead to broken nights' sleep, sometimes for months, occasionally even years. You may find that you have periods of time, coinciding with hormonal fluctuations, when sleep seems repeatedly disturbed. It is unsurprising, then, that you feel tired next day, struggle to work effectively and experience concentration issues. This can lead to you forgetting tasks, missing deadlines and work taking longer than usual. When this happens, it can result in feelings of disappointment in yourself, questioning of your ability and then a lack of confidence. You know you can do the job and do it well, but the outward signs are indicating a potential problem. If you do not communicate carefully to your manager, you risk judgement on your performance, which can lead to further undermining of your confidence. It is much better to raise the issue and seek to address it or find ways of working around problems.

Poor memory can be associated with the menopause but also with ageing. If minor, it is unlikely that you are the only one who has this problem; it's just that most people try to cover it or compensate for it.

You can help yourself by recognising the problem and attempting to address it:

◆ Break tasks down into manageable goals, so that you don't feel overwhelmed with work. Explain to colleagues and managers that this is what you are doing.

◆ Take breaks when due – a change of space, a little fresh air and a break in work is often beneficial.

◆ Reassure work colleagues that the job will be done to your usual high standard, but that you may change the way you do it.

◆ Managers may be more supportive if they can understand the reasons for your behaviour, so be open about how you might change your style of working but still be effective.

◆ If colleagues are aware, they may help you to realise that minor memory slips are unimportant and that, with support, the more important things are not forgotten but just remembered in a different way, e.g. electronic reminders, notes and lists.

◆ If your symptoms mean that you have difficulties doing your job, then it is fair to discuss it with your manager to see if reasonable adjustments can be made to enable you to do the job well. They would much rather you addressed the problem than allowed the situation to worsen.

◆ If you find it hard to speak about this subject with your line manager, seek the advice of another manager in your department or your human resources department, if necessary.

> ### Recommendation
>
> If you are seriously struggling at work because of menopausal symptoms, take time to speak with a manager or with the human resources department to make them aware, while at the same time seeking medical advice to treat the symptoms if appropriate.

Menopausal humour and perceptions

I can see the humour in menopause, but when it's you who are the constant butt of the jokes, it gets very wearing and not at all funny.

We have all seen the menopause jokes – in fact, you have probably made some yourself – but they become tiresome after a while and in the workplace they should be restricted to between friends only. There is no place for the mocking of women going through menopause or of constant reference to it during a working day. It is a serious private matter and, while you might choose to confide in friends at work, or a trusted manager, or even make jokes yourself, it should not become something for public discussion unless you want it to.

In the workplace, there should be a culture of respect, an openness for menopause to be acknowledged without judgement, and a willingness to make minor adjustments to make working life easier, without fanfare and certainly without embarrassment.

I stopped being the one to make the jokes and noticed that others did too.

If you feel that the joke of menopause has worn thin and is becoming irritating and counter-productive, be bold enough to withdraw from the jokes and make it known that you do not find them amusing any more. Your colleagues will take their cue from you; if you joke and treat it lightly, they probably will too. You probably don't mind the odd humorous remark, but frequent reminders or a belittling attitude is unfair.

Talking to managers

Talking to my manager really helped; she was kind and supportive.

I didn't tell my managers because I was worried it would be seen as a weakness.

Should I say it is menopause if my work environment is exacerbating symptoms?

This is an individual choice. It would be good to think that in a modern mixed-gender workplace, you would feel able to mention the 'M' word without embarrassment. In reality, our work colleagues are not always our friends, so discussing personal issues like hormones does not always come naturally. Your manager may be male, younger than you, or simply not very approachable. She may even be a woman who sailed through menopause and thinks everyone else should too.

Times are changing though, and many managers in large corporations will have had 'the menopause talk' at some point in training or in an induction and will have at least some understanding of it. This should result in you being able to raise the subject and make positive suggestions as to how your situation can be improved. Your manager may be embarrassed too, so be clear about what you are hoping for – is it a change of uniform, a change in room temperature, or more major adjustments in working pattern or hours? If the last of these, don't be surprised if you are referred on after your initial discussion, perhaps to the human resources department (HR) or to occupational health (OH), who will be better placed to help you. Larger companies are gradually working to put in place policies and procedures relating to menopause; smaller ones may not. You can find out if there are policies by contacting human resources before having any private discussions about you as an individual.

What if I get nowhere with my manager?

You pluck up the courage to speak to your manager and she, or he, says, or maybe just implies: 'just get on as best you can'. This will not solve the problem or help your work. 'Just getting on' may mean continuing to struggle through without support and adjustments. You may need to approach another manager to get a fruitful discussion. Some organisations have a system in place for 'alternative line manager access' for when you want to discuss something important but don't want your immediate line manager to be aware. This may be a time to use that. If not, contact the HR department: they will have processes in place to help where there is a barrier in communication between managers and employees, whatever the reason.

If I need sick leave because of menopause, do I have to say that is why I am off?

It is unlikely that you will need much time off because of menopause and there is no requirement for you to explicitly disclose menopause as being the reason you are off sick. If you take time off because of debilitating symptoms, fatigue or anxiety, for example, there is no requirement to be specific on the self-certification forms or GP issued 'Fit Notes'. If you take sick leave because you can no longer cope with your workload or do the job effectively because of how you feel, you may decide that this does need to be disclosed because small adjustments may make work life more manageable. From a company perspective, it would be very helpful to know how many women needed time off because of menopausal complaints, but you do not have to disclose unless you want to. If more women reported the actual reason for sick leave, workplaces might find ways to change, as they realise the effect that menopause is having on female employees. It is only too common for 'stress' or 'women's problems' to be described as the reason for leave, when in fact menopausal symptoms may be the root cause.

I am finding it hard to keep doing my job properly, because of symptoms. What are my rights?

Many women make small adjustments to cope with menopause; only a very few need more significant changes or even consider giving up working altogether. Before you reach that stage, seek advice from HR or a union representative or, in a small company, have an honest discussion with managers or bosses. What would it take for you to carry on working productively? Your employer has a responsibility under current Health and Safety Legislation and Gender Equality Legislation to ensure that 'workplaces are suitable for the individuals who work in them' and that the 'health, safety and welfare' of all employees is considered. Organisations cannot just refuse to take seriously small changes that might address your concerns about a particular work environment. Of course, you may be in one of those few jobs where adjustments would alter the manner of the work or impinge on the safety of others, so that has to be taken into account as well. Seek medical help too. If your symptoms are having a severe effect on your work then you may need medical support and getting help as early as possible could mean the difference between being able to continue working or not.

If you are the boss, what can you do?

With an ageing workforce, menopause is a topic that will arise again and again and positively addressing it will promote good health in the workplace and minimise absenteeism. Across the country, women of menopausal age are contributing hugely to company success and to the UK and corporate economy. Menopause can happen at any age, although is most common between the ages of 48 and 55. That means that you may see women much younger who are menopausal and who need support. Don't assume that anyone is 'too young' for menopause or indeed that by a certain age 'surely you are through that by now'. Don't generalise, treat each woman individually, and ask what can be done to support ongoing fruitful work.

Top tips for managers

◆ Menopausal jokes are seldom appropriate at work; when used by women themselves they are probably a defence mechanism to cover embarrassment. Encourage a culture towards women that takes menopause seriously.

◆ Remember that menopausal symptoms are usually short-lived but can last for many years in some women and can be very severely bothersome in a few.

◆ The majority of women will experience some disruption to life and be able to make minor changes to cope at work without consultation with managers. Not every woman going through menopause will have a problem at work.

◆ Consider appointing a 'menopause champion' in the workplace, perhaps providing literature and support without needing to go to line managers.

◆ Educate managers in normal menopause changes and how women might be affected at work. Discuss ways of opening discussions while maintaining respect and dignity.

◆ Consider if you need any policies or guidance for managers.

◆ In the long term, consider a hierarchy of menopausal needs concerning your particular workplace and discuss how as an employer they might be addressed:

Very occasional
job review

Few women – major adjustments with HR/OH
change of hours or specific duties

Some women – support and minor adjustments
perhaps fans, uniform allowances

All women – information and education
through well-being events and open discussion

Why can't they just get on with it?

Some men and women are heard to say this. Well, that is exactly what most women do. All women go through menopause if they live long enough, less than half seek medical help, and around a quarter have symptoms that they describe as moderate to severe. Some women will get no symptoms at all. It is the exceptions, the worst affected women, those with severe symptoms or particularly long-lasting ones, who will need employer support. In a Nuffield Health Survey in 2014, 10 per cent of more than 3,000 women reported that they had seriously considered giving up work. Most women in this situation will seek medical help if needed and the time for work adjustments will be short. It is very rare that women need long-term significant work adjustments, but when they do, employer support is vital.

Is everything down to hormones?

'Menopause' should not become a label for anything that happens to affect midlife women. They can still get illnesses and medical conditions that are nothing to do with hormones. It may take a while for women to acknowledge this and it may take a little time to get medical help as even clinicians tend to blame the menopause for everything that happens to a woman around the age of 50. It can be a slow process to reach a different diagnosis when menopausal symptoms are featuring so strongly.

There is no legislation specifically related to menopause, but it does come under employment law through other legislation. The health, safety and welfare at work regulations can be applied to this issue, and the manager or employer who ignores menopause and its impact may be at risk of breach of these rules.

Communication, support and sensitivity with employees are essential in order to achieve a better understanding of the menopause and how it affects the individual. Perhaps it is time to have a section in the staff handbook relating to how menopause may affect work and how to access support if needed. Occupational health departments can make themselves aware of local resources or clinics where help can be found if so desired. The next chapter discusses how to access support. For some women, it may be occupational health staff who help them navigate their way through the NHS in order to find the appropriate help. Employers may want to use some of the resources in the final section to compile literature for staff, either as short leaflets or as web-based materials on staff intranet pages. Having such information easily accessible to all staff, not just those with menopause, encourages an awareness about the topic that will be of benefit to the whole organisation.

chapter 8

Seeking help at menopause

I knew I wanted help; getting it was harder than I expected.

There is so little time at appointments – where do you begin?

I don't want just to be handed a prescription; I want much more information than that.

Menopause is not an illness; you may not need help at all when it occurs. If you don't get symptoms that are too troublesome and you take steps to maintain good health, the chances are that you will not need medical or any other type of help as you go through the transition. Unless it happens early, menopause is natural and the medical approach is not appropriate for everyone. The consequences of menopause, like hot flushes, night sweats, tiredness, poor concentration and everything we discussed in Chapter 1, may, however, lead you to seek help or support. You may want to discuss your symptoms and check that they are actually menopause-related and not something else. You may have risk factors for diseases in your family that lead you to a discussion about what steps you should take to avoid certain conditions, and menopause may be the time to do this. Perhaps your mum had osteoporosis and you want to minimise your own risk. You may be at the point where your symptoms are really affecting your home, social and work life, and you may want to explore treatment options. You may be going through menopause under the age of 40, or as a result of cancer treatments, or having made the difficult choice to have risk-reducing surgery that has rendered you meno-pausal suddenly and at a young age. Any one of these might send you looking for help and advice – so where can you go?

The media – newspapers, magazines and television

Headlines seem to swing from one way to another.

Why no good news stories on menopause?

The subject of menopause and in particular HRT is very popular with the press. Women's magazines and daily newspapers all cover the topic, and more recently there has been television coverage as well. Some of this coverage is accurate, informative and educational; some is not. It can be interesting to read stories about individual women and how they cope, but very often a piece is written to emphasise just one aspect of menopause, which may promote a view that is unbal-anced or even, occasionally, prejudiced. Some journal-ists have their own strong opinions on menopause, and that is sometimes reflected in the writing. Some will have researched the topic and will present current thinking in a balanced way, but others may not, and advice might be out of date or simply incomplete. If you see headlines in the newspaper about HRT, they are most likely to be negative: that is what makes good headlines. Don't stop any treatments based on headlines in the media. Read with interest but check it out and if you read something that makes you worry, speak to your doctor.

Websites and books

I found it so useful to read the information at my own pace and in an easy to read format.

I found conflicting advice from different places; I got more confused and more anxious as I read.

Probably the first place you will turn to is the internet and using the computer in the privacy of your home means that you can spend many hours looking up menopause and all the associated symptoms, treatments and advice. Much of what you will find will be helpful and medically accurate, but lots will not be; how do you know what to trust and what to discard? You will find many, many stories from women sharing their experience of menopause, some of which you will find inspiring, some scary, and some a little astonishing: it is surprising what some people will share online. You might end up accessing information from anywhere in the world, written by anyone in the world. Writers of books (including this one) are influenced by their own knowledge, understanding and, to some extent, their personal values, as they explore an area of health and its management. Looking behind the website and behind the author, by researching the background, qualifications and credibility of the writer, will help you to sift out that which might be unhelpful.

How to find a good website

1 Is it accurate?

Find out who is writing the pages. Look at the 'about us' section. What are their credentials for writing about menopause? Does the page refer to scientific reports or data, and explain it in language that is easy to understand? Check several websites and see if advice is consistent across sites. Look for sites written by those working in the field of menopause that supports the information given with links to government guidance and to reference materials. Is it just a site offering someone's opinion, or does it demonstrate a base of clinical research? Is the advice relevant to the UK and UK clinical practice?

2 Is it biased?

Who pays for the website? A site supported by a commercial company might be very accurate, or it could be a place to sell products – take a careful look for advertising. Be wary of 'miracle cures' or quick links to buy products. On medical websites there will be a clear distinction between advertising and information, whereas a commercial page might be more blurred, mentioning only their product as a solution. On medical websites, there will be a clear notice indicating that products advertised are just that – adverts, not endorsements.

3 *Is it up to date?*

Medical information changes fast and there should be a date on the website of the most recent update, hopefully in the last five years. If not, ask yourself, how do I know this is still accurate? The date indicates that the information has been checked, even if there was no need for change.

4 *Be wary*

If you read personal stories, remember that every woman is different and you are an individual. It can be helpful to read about other's experiences around menopause, but be aware that that is what they are – personal stories from anyone around the world.

Books / articles

Similar principles as those for websites apply to books and articles except that it is much harder to keep these updated. So check the date of publication and ask yourself: is that recent enough to be still relevant? Is the topic one that might be changing rapidly or is reasonably constant? Most general information about menopause and its effects will hold true for some years and an old book is not necessarily irrelevant. Over five to ten years, HRT evidence might change quite significantly, so, if you are looking for accurate information about treatments, look for a recently published book. Look at the author – do they have experience and education in this area? Are they qualified to write in their chosen style? Does the book aim to educate, in which case you want the author to be knowledgeable and qualified, or is it a book about personal experience, in which the author shares their story in order to broaden understanding but doesn't aim to give advice? Both types have their place, so decide which you want.

Menopause groups and peer support

It was so helpful to realise that other women are going through the same thing – no one talks about it.

Until I joined a group, it [menopause] *felt like a taboo word no one wanted to talk about.*

Most of these are set up by enthusiastic women who want to help others because they found it difficult to access information and advice. Some are led by therapists or life coaches, others by medical practitioners, and some by women with no health qualifications but a good understanding of the changes that occur during menopause. It can be an excellent way to share an understanding of menopause and realise that you are not alone in your experiences. Leaders or facilitators will often be very knowledgeable and can point you towards the right type of help. They are not usually qualified practitioners, although they may be, and advice is likely to be general rather than medical and specific to you.

Look at their credentials so that you know what to expect from the group and check if anything is being marketed alongside – hidden advertising.

Medical help

Your GP

My doctor was sympathetic, but didn't know where to start.

I had under ten minutes – how do you cover it all in ten minutes?

If you want HRT or other medical help, your first step will be to discuss it with your general practitioner (GP). With a little homework beforehand, you can help yourself get the best from the appointment by considering the following.

◆ Which GP? In many practices, there will be one or more GPs who have a particular interest in women's health and so will be most knowledgeable. Others might be more knowledgeable in other conditions, like diabetes, asthma or children's conditions. Perhaps ask the receptionist as they often have a good idea about who might be best for you to see, or check the practice handbook for each doctor's area of special interest.

◆ Think ahead – are you looking mainly for diagnosis and reassurance or are you looking for medical treatment? Your GP will be led by your opening questions, so be clear from the outset what you hope to get from the consultation.

◆ Plan your questions – there may not be time for as many as you would like, so think about two or three key questions, particularly ones that apply only to you – personal, relevant and meaningful.

◆ Do some preparation – get a general understanding of menopause and its treatment options before you go so that your questions can be specific and concise.

◆ Don't be surprised if you are asked to come back for a further appointment and are given leaflets or website addresses to look at. This may be frustrating but your GP wants to be sure that you are fully informed before starting any treatment and this is one way of doing so – making you do even more homework.

◆ Remember that you may not need any tests (see Chapter 1), so don't be disappointed if you are not offered any.

Sexual health services

It was natural to talk about HRT to the person who advised me about contraception in my late forties – it made sense as they needed to fit together.

You may already be attending a sexual health service to discuss contraception. Doctors and nurses who work in these clinics (called CASH – Contraceptive and Sexual Health) often work widely in women's health and can advise about menopause too. There is an overlap in services between menopause and contraception and the time comes when you may need both, so speak to your sexual health doctor if you want further advice about menopause. They will also know of other menopause services in your area, should you need them, and can make recommendations to your GP based on what you discuss.

Specialist menopause clinics

It was such a relief to talk to someone who really understands the nuances of HRT and could find one that was right for me. I had tried a few already ...

The menopause clinic gave me what my lovely GP couldn't – time and expert knowledge about a complex case.

Specialist menopause clinics are few and far between. Not all areas will have one and you may have to do some research in order to find one in your area. Menopause specialists are often but not always doctors and may work in a variety of settings. You may find one in your local gynaecology clinic, in a GP practice, a sexual health service, or attached to another clinic, like endocrinology (hormone clinic). They might be in a hospital-based service or a community-based clinic and might work alone or as part of a team. Specialists will receive referrals from other clinicians and have a wealth of knowledge and experience in menopause and its treatments. The aim of a specialist is not to see all women, but to be available to those women whose medical history, HRT history, or personal circumstances make their case just a bit more complicated. Usually, you will need a referral from your GP. You can look at a list of clinics on the website www.menopausematters. co.uk (see the Resources chapter).

You may not need a specialist; in many cases, your GP will be very able to advise and treat your symptoms. Your GP may consider referring you to a specialist, if there is one near you, in the following circumstances:

◆ You are under the age of 40, and diagnosis and management is unclear, or you need extra support through the diagnosis of premature ovarian insufficiency (see Chapter 5).

◆ You are about to become menopausal due to planned surgery and want to discuss how you will deal with health and symptoms afterwards. For example, you may be opting for risk-reducing oophorectomy (see Chapter 5) or you may have surgery or medical treatment to treat cancer, which will put you into menopause (see Chapter 6).

◆ You may have tried several HRTs and been unable to find one that suits you.

◆ You may have been told that there are medical reasons to avoid HRT, but you still have bothersome symptoms. A specialist can discuss your options with you, suggest other ways of managing symptoms and sometimes suggest ways of using HRT that are low-risk, despite your medical situation.

Private clinics

I am willing to pay, just to get the help I need.

There seem to be a lot of private 'specialists': how do I choose?

If you decide you want to be seen privately for treatment of your menopausal symptoms, you may not be covered by any health insurance plan, although it is worth asking the question of your insurance company. Bear in mind that you need to consider not just the initial consultation fee, but also any tests or investigations that might be necessary and the cost of an ongoing private prescription if you take one. Going private gives you:

◆ Choice of where and when to be seen

◆ Selection of specialist

◆ Fast access to an appointment.

Before choosing a private menopause appointment, do your research:

◆ Does the practitioner regularly see and advise women on menopause? (You may notice that they do this on the NHS.)

◆ What are their qualifications and special interests? You can ask if they have registered with the British Menopause Society (the UK professional organisation) as a menopause specialist.

◆ Do they prescribe treatments that are regulated by the MHRA (Medicines and Healthcare Regulatory Authority)? If not, find out what treatments are offered and how they are regulated.

◆ Seek a recommendation. Your GP or practice nurse might be able to help.

Treatment or not: weighing up the options

I just want someone to tell me what to do; that's what I go to the doctor for.

Unlike many areas of medicine, there is not always a clear answer as to whether or not to have treatment for menopausal symptoms – it really is often up to you. You may get a strong recommendation, especially if you are young, but ultimately it is often your choice – treat symptoms or not? You will want to gather information, ask questions and make the decision that is right for you. Somebody else in a similar situation may make a different choice. In making a choice to take treatment, you might want to consider:

◆ Potential benefit – which symptoms might improve and by how much? (See Chapter 4 on HRT.)

◆ Base rate risks – what is known about the treatment and the general risk it might carry to a population of women using it?

◆ Perceived personal risk – think about your personal and medical history: what is the risk to you? This is 'individualising risk'. A skilled clinician will help you do this.

◆ Personal values – you are unique, and your acceptance of risk will differ to someone else's. If you have known a loved one with breast cancer, you will have one view, if you know someone with fractures due to osteoporosis, your opinion might be different.

You might have ideas about what is 'natural' or not; and being able to carry on working may be important to you, or it may not be. How you cope with your symptoms is unique to you. These personal values will vary between women and are neither right nor wrong; they simply make you who you are and will influence your decision about treatments.

Whether you see someone privately or under the NHS, your healthcare professional should talk with you about your menopause experience, explain any tests that might be necessary (or, indeed, why they are not required), offer ways of managing symptoms with and without HRT, and offer treatment if that is what you want. If treatment is offered, you need to be confident that you have been treated as an individual and that the treatment is appropriate for you. Ideally, you will have an opportunity to discuss the risk of future disease such as osteoporosis and heart disease and how you might limit your risk for these conditions (see Chapter 2). You might want to talk about contraception – what to use and when to stop. Any treatment should come with a plan for follow-up and advice about any potential side effects. You might want to ask:

◆ What are my treatment options and what do you recommend?

◆ What are the risks of the treatment for me and what side effects might I get?

◆ How long do you suggest treatment for?

◆ How often do I need to return for monitoring?

Having had a good discussion I can now make the right decision for me.

You might decide that you don't need medical treatment after all: you feel reassured, have received good information, and with that knowledge decide against it. If you do not get the information that you need or feel you do not have the understanding and knowledge to make a good decision, seek further help.

Use the information in this book, and the websites and organisations recommended in the Resources section, to equip yourself with understanding, and then prepare the questions you still have and ask your doctor. That way you can use the time in the consultation to your individual benefit.

Resources

About menopause

Daisy Network
www.daisynetwork.org.uk
Online support network for women with premature
ovarian insufficiency. UK site, open to all, with access
to clinical specialists through live chat sessions.

Manage my menopause
Managemymenopause.co.uk

Advice tailored to you through interactive questions.
Developed by UK clinicians.

Menopause Matters
www.menopausematters.co.uk
Comprehensive clinician-led UK website about all
things menopause. Includes an online forum and shop.

NHS Choices
www.nhs.uk/Conditions/Menopause/Pages/
Introduction.aspx
Menopause pages within a general NHS information
site.

UK NICE Guidance 2015

Diagnosis and management of menopause.
www.nice.org.uk/guidance/ng23
Information for women and health professionals.

Women's Health Concern

www.womens-health-concern.org
Patient arm of the British Menopause Society, with information on many women's health topics. WHC has a nurse-led advice centre you may contact by email or telephone (small charge).

After cancer

BRCA

www.brcaumbrella.ning.com
Membership support for those affected by BRCA. Some detailed surgical pictures.

Clarissa Foster, *Understanding BRCA – What you need to know*, Hammersmith Health Books, 2017.

Breast Cancer Care

www.breastcancercare.org.uk
Information and support for women who have had breast cancer – useful section on menopausal symptoms with breast cancer treatments.

Cancer Research UK

www.cancerresearchuk.org
Information and research on all types of cancers.

Eve Appeal

www.eveappeal.org.uk

UK charity dedicated to raising awareness and funding research into the five gynaecological cancers – ovarian, cervical, womb, vaginal and vulval. 'Ask Eve' is an opportunity to speak to a specialist nurse by telephone.

Jo's Cervical Cancer Trust

www.jostrust.org.uk

UK charity dedicated to women affected by cervical cancer and cervical abnormalities. Useful section on early menopause after cervical cancer.

Macmillan Cancer Support

www.macmillan.org.uk

Information and support after cancer, including fact sheets on reducing risk of complications after early menopause.

Ovacome

www.ovacome.org.uk

UK charity with information and support about ovarian cancer, including access to free telephone advice with a specialist nurse.

Health topics

Adoption

www.first4adoption.org.uk

British Heart Foundation

www.bhf.org.uk

There is a section on menopause and heart disease.

Contraception

www.fpa.org.uk

Help, advice and information on issues relating to sexual health, including choices of contraception.

Exercise and weight management

www.nhs.uk/livewell

Excellent tips and advice for increasing exercise and maintaining a healthy weight.

Fertility

Human fertilisation and embryology authority
www.hfea.gov.uk

As well as being a regulatory organisation, the HFEA offers support and information about all aspects of fertility treatments.

FRAX – fracture risk assessment tool

www.shef.ac.uk

Select the calculation tool to calculate ten-year risk of osteoporotic facture. Speak to your doctor if you fall in the red or orange risk area.

National Osteoporosis Society

www.nos.org.uk

UK charity dedicated to eradicating osteoporosis and promoting bone health. Fact sheets and tips, including calcium calculator for foods and nurse helpline.

Pelvic floor exercise and bladder health
www.bladderandbowel.org

RELATE
www.relate.org.uk
Relationship support for all, offering counselling and information, as well as practical tips and guides to help you manage common relationship issues. Telephone, email and chat counselling available (fee for some services).

Slimming World
www.slimmingworld.co.uk

Stop smoking advice
www.nhs.uk/smokefree/help-and-advice
Tips, advice and resources to help you stop smoking.

Surrogacy
www.surrogacyuk.org

Weightwatchers
www.weightwatchers.com/uk

Therapies

Association of Reflexologists
www.aor.org.uk

British Acupuncture Council
www.acupuncture.org.uk

Cognitive Behavioural Therapy (CBT)

Myra Hunter and Melanie Smith, *Managing hot flushes and night sweats – A cognitive behavioural self-help guide to the menopause*, Routledge, 2013.

British Association for Behavioural and Cognitive Psychotherapies
www.babcp.co.uk
All about CBT, how to find a therapist, what to expect and more.

Fact sheet (full version of the text adapted in Chapter 3 of this book)
www.womens-health-concern.org

Counselling

www.counselling-directory.org.uk
Information and resources about counselling, including what to expect and how to access professionals.

Institute of Psychosexual Medicine

www.ipm.org.uk

Psychosexual therapy

www.cosrt.org.uk
Find a therapist, useful tips and information about sex and relationships.

Menopause and work

Faculty of Occupational Medicine
www.fom.ac.uk/health-at-work-2/information-for-employers/dealing-with-health-problems-in-the-workplace/advice-on-the-menopause
Guidance for employers with tips, statistics and useful tools to raise awareness.

Several unions have produced documentation around menopause at work. These are examples:

NASUWT (teachers' union)
www.nasuwt.org.uk
Managing the menopause in the workplace.

RCN (nurses' union)
www.rcn.org.uk
Menopause and work – guidance for RCN representatives.

Trades Union Congress
www.tuc.org.uk/workplace-issues
Advice on supporting women through menopause in the workplace.

UNISON
www.unison.org.uk
Menopause Factsheet.

Want to contact me? You can do so through my website: www.kathyabernethy.com

Acknowledgements

When I first started working in a menopause clinic in the mid 1980s, even though I was too young to fully appreciate the effects of the menopause on women, I began to get some understanding of how great an impact this natural life event can have. Over the years, and having worked in several menopause clinics, my knowledge has been deepened by the many women of all ages who have shared their menopause journeys with me and have contributed to my knowledge and understanding.

I am proud to have been part of the British Menopause Society since its inception, and I wish to thank all my colleagues, past and present, for their ongoing support and enthusiasm as we work towards providing education, information and guidance on health issues relating to menopausal health. I particularly want to thank Joan Pitkin, consultant gynaecologist, for her never-ceasing encouragement. My thanks too to Myra Hunter, emeritus professor of clinical health psychology, King's College London, for allowing the adaptation of her resources on cognitive behavioural therapy.

Thanks are due to my husband, Mark, and children, Josh, Elli and Charlotte, who have patiently listened to me over the years getting more and more enthusiastic about menopause, not a subject teens usually discuss.

Thanks too to Sue Wing, Jane Woyka and Dani Singer, who read drafts of sections of the book and helped shape its final form.

Finally, thank you to Rebecca Gray and her team at Profile Books, for their encouragement and advice in producing this book.

Index